sleepwalker

THE MYSTERIOUS MAKINGS AND RECOVERY

OF A SOMNAMBULIST

KATHLEEN FRAZIER

Foreword by **DR. MARK MAHOWALD**

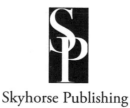

Skyhorse Publishing

Skyhorse Publishing books may be purchased in bulk at special discounts for sales promotion, corporate gifts, fund-raising, or educational purposes. Special editions can also be created to specifications. For details, contact the Special Sales Department, Skyhorse Publishing, 307 West 36th Street, 11th Floor, New York, NY 10018 or info@skyhorsepublishing.com.

Skyhorse® and Skyhorse Publishing® are registered trademarks of Skyhorse Publishing, Inc.®, a Delaware corporation.

Visit our website at www.skyhorsepublishing.com.

10 9 8 7 6 5 4 3 2 1

Library of Congress Cataloging-in-Publication Data is available on file.

Cover design by Brian Peterson

Print ISBN: 978-1-63450-235-1
Ebook ISBN: 978-1-5107-0070-3

Printed in the United States of America

Have mercy on my memory,
I sleepwalked through most of it.

CONTENTS

FOREWORD

THE DOCTOR'S OPINION

Kathleen Frazier's powerful and beautifully written memoir successfully fills a huge void by providing helpful and valuable information on sleepwalking and sleep terrors by someone who is able to elucidate what these poorly understood phenomena are, how they are misinterpreted, and, most importantly, the extent to which they may greatly affect one's behavior and well-being.

For centuries, sleepwalking and sleep terrors were believed to be caused by diverse and usually undesirable phenomena such as acting out repressed waking desires, "devil or demon possession," or psychiatric disease. One of the original terms for sleepwalking, *moonstruck*, brings to mind fictional creatures from gothic horror such as werewolves. Until recently, no effective treatments had been developed. It is highly likely that a good number of church-sanctioned exorcisms were, and still are, being performed for this medical condition.

Only recently has the underlying neurophysiology been explained. We now know that during sleepwalking and sleep terrors, the part of the brain that generates very complex behaviors is awake, while the part of the brain that normally monitors what we do and lays down memories of what we have done is asleep. This condition leaves the brain in a mixed wake/sleep state, capable of generating wild behaviors without conscious awareness and therefore without culpability. It is not known what causes this "state dissociation" (a mixture of wakefulness and sleep), but importantly, and contrary to popular opinion, it is not related to significant underlying psychiatric or psychological problems.

About one-third of American adults report having had an episode of sleepwalking. Yet sleepwalkers and those suffering from sleep terrors typically hesitate to seek medical attention. Still laboring under old ideas, they fear being told the episodes are due to psychiatric illness, and the nature of the episodes is often embarrassing. A potentially violent or injurious episode often leads to evaluation. Yet effective medical treatments are now available—actually a number of them—such as medication and hypnosis. The key is finding a sleep medicine professional experienced in the diagnosis and management of sleepwalking and sleep terrors.

Sleepwalking and sleep terrors affected every part of Ms. Frazier's life. They put her safety, her very life, at risk and threatened the safety of those close to her. *Sleepwalker: The Mysterious Makings and Recovery of a Somnambulist* is an accurate and fact-filled account, offering hope to those suffering from sleepwalking or sleep terrors, their family members, and also to the professionals who work with them. More, her courage in honestly sharing her fascinating and moving story will appeal to all—sleep being such an intimate and mysterious part of our human condition.

Mark W. Mahowald, MD
Former Director of the Minnesota Regional Sleep Disorders Center
Retired Professor, Dept. of Neurology, University of MN Medical School
Adjunct Professor, Department of Psychiatry and Behavioral Sciences, Stanford University
Consultant, Sleep Forensics Associates

My long nightgown twisted around my ankles. I'd always hated that trapped feeling. I turned from side to side on the moldy couch in a ridiculous effort to get comfortable. The springs of the sofa were nocturnal animals. They poised patiently, waiting for the exact instant when my body surrendered to sleep so they could pounce up and bite me. I spent this particular night in the enormous living room of Bob and Jane's apartment to avoid the smell of paint drying in my rented postage stamp of a bedroom. Deep blue had been my color choice, having read it could calm the nerves.

A month shy of twenty-nine, I was an aspiring actress resigned to communal living, one of several boarders in the rambling flat located on the Upper West Side of Manhattan. My landlords were middle-aged Bohemians, writers, filmmakers. He was a philanderer. I'd played a Wild West saloon whore in a music video they'd made for a jazz saxophonist, which is how we became roommates. Their labyrinth halls led to disheveled rooms, some of which overlooked the Hudson with breathtaking views through windows left wide open in the unbearable summer heat.

Excruciatingly shy, I barely knew the names of the other tenants who wandered the hallways en route from their bedrooms to one of the many bathrooms. Some of them hardly left their quarters. Others came and went quickly, keeping odd hours. My room was in the back, off the kitchen, with a small, dirty window that faced an airshaft. Once the maid's room, it included a closet-sized bathroom with toilet and sink. I hated having to shower or bathe in one of the larger bathrooms, shared with strangers.

If sharing a bathroom unnerved me, the idea of bunking down in an open, common space, through which one or more of them would pass during the course of the evening, horrified me. I especially cringed at the idea of Bob creeping past me in the middle of the night upon his return from a liaison.

Despite condemning myself as juvenile, I'd plugged in my angel night-light nearby. I wore my best nightgown, too—lightweight and sleeveless but modest. Even in the dark, appearances mattered to me. It was the prettiest shade of rose pink, my mother's favorite flower. She was Catherine Rose and I wore it in her honor. It was August 6, 1988, and would have been her sixty-eighth birthday had she not died of cancer a little more than a year earlier. I'd been attending a bereavement group at CancerCare the whole time, and it seemed to me that my grief should have eased after the one-year anniversary of my mom's death. Instead it weighed heavier than ever.

Green glow-in-the-dark numbers on my radio alarm clock flipped in slow motion.

I turned on a reading lamp and the sudden light sent a cockroach scampering across the hardwood floor beneath a huge, discarded pile of newspapers. How would I ever fall asleep with the fear of the disgusting creatures crawling all over me at my most vulnerable?

I banished the thought by picking up C. S. Lewis's The Screwtape Letters *about a senior demon's counsel to his nephew on how to damn a man. I read until my eyes felt heavy. I let them close, resting the Devil's letters against the thump, thump, thump of my heart. Blood pulsed through my ears. As a kid, I'd listened to that dreadful sound for what seemed like hours as I tried to fall asleep. Nicknamed Kitten by my family, I was a born scaredy-cat, afraid of bedtime from the start. When I was quite small, I shared a room with my brother, Danny, two years my senior. An impressionable Catholic school girl, I found it easy to believe his good-night stories. If we stepped off our beds, some creature would drag us under, the Devil or one of his helpers, rats, snakes, take your pick.*

I realized, as I was about to drift off on the lumpy sofa, that these were not the most soothing bedtime thoughts. Reaching to turn out the light, I changed my mind and left it on. I must have fallen asleep then. I don't know for how long.

DEAD TO THE WORLD

Once upon a time, long before my family reported episodes of sleepwalking and sleep terrors, there was the feeling of impending doom. Going to bed always carried with it a kind of animal fear. The despair I felt at leaving this world behind, of separating myself from the people I loved, was all-consuming. I am certain of these feelings, yet my earliest memories of sleep are watery, elusive. What do I remember—and what were stories retold to me by my four older siblings and parents over and over until they laid a track in my mind that mimicked memory? When was I awake and when was I asleep?

First there was the deep, dreamless slumber of a toddler, fingers curled and lips bowed. The complete surrender of physical exhaustion. Then the shock of unearthly screams and confusion. Panic, as I struggled from tucked blankets and fumbled for my crib panel just in time to see my mother fly past my doorway. A banshee in a nightie. Why was she fleeing? Who was taking her from me? Suddenly, the whole house came to life. My father's voice boomed from the other end of the hall—"Oh my God, Kate, no!"—and footsteps thundered down the stairway as my older siblings Patty, Mary Ann, and Billy ran from the second floor. I burst out crying and Danny, who was probably five, was out of his bed and at my side in an instant, hanging on to my crib's railing, howling along with me.

A banshee is a female spirit in Gaelic folklore whose appearance or wailing often presages a death in the family. And so, sleeping posed a fatal prospect from the very start in the Frazier house. We didn't have a word to describe my mother's violent nocturnal wanderings beyond *nightmares*. Very, very bad nightmares. We avoided discussion of things that went bump in the night. We never used the word *sleepwalker* to describe her; it sounded too crazy. The terms *night terror/sleep terror* were not around. There were no sleep clinics in the 1960s.

I was left alone in the dark to unpack my mother's fearsome episodes. I'm uncertain the extent to which I was traumatized by her severely disturbed sleep and whether somewhere in my little girl mind I worried it would happen to me.

My father was a phantom of a different sort. Insomnia left him up all hours, wandering about, lost in his own home.

One winter's night, when I had finally graduated from the crib to a twin, I woke to see fingers of light reaching down the otherwise darkened hallway. I don't know how long I lay awake, unused to my new mobility and fretting over whether I should sneak from my big-girl bed to investigate. Finally, I tiptoed in my footed pajamas toward the living room, teddy bear in hand, floorboards creaking, and imagined ghosts released with every footfall.

There sat my father, surrounded by a haze of cigar smoke, perched on the edge of his La-Z-Boy recliner, footrest tucked away. He was leaning over a thousand-piece puzzle spread before him on our card table. He peered through black-rimmed bifocals, the butt of his stogie burned unattended in a glass ashtray. It seemed he'd never notice me, afraid as I was to make a peep. Would I be a welcome relief to his lonely night or would my interruption anger him? My mother had used the term *like walking on eggshells* to describe being around my father, and this night I imagined the living room floor strewn with empty, cracked shells between us. His balding head rested in his hands. His eyelids drooped and I thought for a minute that he'd fallen asleep, sitting up like that.

"Daddy," I whispered.

"Kitten, what are you doing out of bed?"

Met with his gentle voice, my whole body relaxed.

The puzzle was almost finished and he gestured for me to take a look. I saw giants' faces stuck in stone, and it frightened me. Years later, I would realize it had been an image of Mount Rushmore. But in that moment, I covered my eyes. He pulled me onto his skinny lap to comfort me. I placed my head against his steady heart.

"Why are you up, Daddy?"

"Keeping guard, Kitten."

"From the bogeyman?"

"I got the worry gene, that's all. And it looks like you do too." He rubbed his thumb between my eyebrows in an effort to erase my furrowed brow.

My parents were like cars speeding out of control, brakes slammed on, spinning wildly in an effort to right themselves against the pressure of generations of drink, mental illness, and resultant sleepless nights. Both had been Depression kids, raised in the city of Albany, New York, and both had survived alcoholic fathers.

Although my father lost his dad when he was only eleven, he'd been anchored to this world by his Irish mother, a stalwart icebox of a widow who worked days as a domestic servant and nights cleaning offices to keep her family together. I've no idea when she slept. Even worse was my mother's childhood. In addition to having an absentee father, her mom had been in and out of psychiatric hospitals with schizophrenia. Often, she had no parent to hold her hand, to tether her to this world. Aunties saved her and her siblings from orphanages. She was a waif seeking the warmth of the public library where she felt safe enough to fall asleep.

Once grown, Mom found independence in the WAVES (Women Accepted for Voluntary Emergency Service). My parents met after World War II. William Francis Frazier had been a sergeant in the army and had seen enough action to keep anyone up nights. Catherine Rose was a plump beauty with skin so soft we called her the smooth-faced lady.

Dad inherited the drinking problem. The Irish euphemism was *he likes his drink*. He took the pledge several times, a Catholic's commitment to sobriety, but slipped repeatedly. They had three children within three years. Eight years later, Danny was born. Eventually, Mom took her Irish triplets and the baby and left Dad. Eventually, he found support with men and women who helped each other stay sober. Mom returned and he put down the drink for good. He got sober around the time I was born, breaking the many-linked chain of alcoholism that had bound our family as far back as our stories stretched.

My parents bought a Cape Cod in a small development in a suburb of Albany. Ours was a blue-collar family with a devoted, stay-at-home mother and a strapping father, lean and strong from loading kegs of Schaefer beer on and off the delivery truck and down treacherous steps to barroom cellars. He'd gone bald early. My mother said it was from all the stress of the war, not to mention his drinking days—he only had a quarter of his stomach after his surgery for ulcers.

It was almost as though we were two families. Patty, Mary Ann, and Billy, three little steps of stairs my mother used to say, then eight years passed before Danny and, two years later, me. As the youngest of five, I entered the wreckage of my parents' past, the chaos of early sobriety, and their sheer exhaustion.

While growing up, my mother often proudly recounted this story about how she'd managed my toddler sleep. Every time she told it, my heart plummeted. I felt ashamed of and confused by my sorrow in the face of her sunny pride.

My parents and four older siblings went on their customary two-week summer vacation and left me behind to stay with relatives.

Mom said it was not an uncommon practice during the early sixties with so many babies booming, but search as I may I have never found another family who did this. Was I a bad girl? A troublemaker? Aunt Helen and Uncle Harold had nine kids, and everyone laughed at the part of the story when my mom's sister slapped my face for *I don't know what* and how I refused to speak to her during the rest of my stay. This proved my wickedness and I laughed too, but it was right about then when my heart began its heavy journey southward. Next, Mom would say that by the time my family returned, they were strange to me. *Strange to me?* What could she possibly have meant by that expression? Tears of anger threatened every time I heard it. I'd even bite the inside of my cheek to prevent them from betraying the ugly emotion. That first night back with my brood, I cried and cried in my crib and not just for an hour, or even for a few.

I wept all the night through.

Mom said she'd read in Dr. Spock's baby book that if a parent goes to a child who is crying inconsolably in her crib, the child would be spoiled.

The next morning, our neighbor from two houses up the block came knocking at our door. "What's wrong with the baby?" she asked, worried about my well-being.

My mother was peeved at our neighbor's interference and pleased by her own resolve. I have no idea what she told the woman.

I'd been left twice, first to my callous aunt and then in my hard crib, and everyone seemed to find it hilarious. With each retelling of the tale, my heart fell further until I imagined myself a heartless girl, it having sunk straight through the soles of my feet to disappear past our hard-wood floors and beyond our cemented basement. I imagined it buried in the concrete of our foundation while I walked hollow-chested. I was smarter without it. I became the good girl. I grew watchful, wary, ever-vigilant. I would have stayed up all night if my body let me.

According to the story, I never cried again at bedtime. I slept deeply. Dead to the world. What Mommy didn't know is that it took hours for me to fall asleep, worrying in bed over all my name-less fears. I despised one particular bedtime prayer, yet found myself whispering repeatedly:

Now I lay me down to sleep
I pray the Lord my soul to keep
If I should die before I wake
I pray the Lord my soul to take

Soon Mom began boasting, "Kathy's so quiet, you wouldn't even know she was here." It is a particular vantage point, the youngest of many siblings. If I had been a superhero, I would have chosen invisibility as my power. And in a way, I had done just that, making no waves during the day but always wary of tsunamis at night.

Sleep is nothing if not mysterious. A practice in letting go. A measure of trust. Every evening each of us, all alone and in the light of our own circumstances, surrenders to sleep. Or tries to.

Before I started sleepwalking or having night terrors, I experienced recurring nightmares like most kids do. Mine were of a less common theme than being chased by monsters or toys turned menacing. They reflected a real incident that took place when I was three.

We were visiting my Great Aunt Kathleen at her cabin on the shore of an upstate lake. It was a small body of icy water, but to me it was as wide as the sea and as curious as it was foreboding. I was hopping about in shallow waters, the squish of silt between my toes, a welcome relief from the sharp stones I made effort to avoid. I also hated the long sheaths of weeds that undulated and wrapped around my little-girl legs.

Danny suddenly appeared before me, an explosion of splashing arms, his face contorted in an impish grin, his dark eyes wide against his pale skin. "Watch out for water snakes!"

Maybe those were not long strands of grass that waved murky and suspect through the green water. Algae conspired. My heart beat faster as I turned to face the shore, which now seemed miles away. I could hear laughter through the screen door from the bungalow beyond. I must have taken one giant step back instead of forward and the bottom was gone.

I breathed in the lake, sinking deeper like in a dream. Everything was slow motion and dark and cold. I felt what I was sure were snakes, hundreds of snakes, swirling around my ankles, then my legs and body, pulling me under—then blankness.

But my head popped up like a jack-in-the-box. Water splashed wildly beneath my frantic hands. I saw the blur of green trees and Aunt Kathleen's cabin, such a pretty pastel with darker trim.

And I saw panic on Danny's big-boy face. He hollered for help.

Billy had been sunning his golden-haired self on the floating dock when the commotion caught his attention. He sat up and called out, "Kathy!" Fear rang in his voice. Then he dove in, my Tarzan, to save me. Down I went a second time, the shivering cold surrounding me. My ears were full of water. I saw Billy again, this time beneath the surface. His face twisted, as if he were crying.

A long time seemed to pass until I opened my eyes to see the camp's wood-beamed ceiling and sinister, dark circles—faces of ghosts staring down at me. Maybe I was dead or in the scene from *The Wizard of Oz* when Dorothy lands back in Kansas. My fingers were blue and I heard the chatter of my baby teeth.

I found myself in a bed that was not my own, wrapped in a blanket. I pulled the satin trim to my chin, for safety's sake. My father's cousin, Father Joe, leaned over me. He patted my forehead with his priestly hand. "We almost lost you, little one."

Billy, age twelve, had saved my life.

After the near drowning, I suffered dark nightmares of great bodies of water. They'd appear out of nowhere, wash over me, envelop me, or prevent me from passing to where I knew I must go. But just as often, it would be Billy's face I'd dream disappearing, sinking into watery depths. It was excruciating. I was powerless to help him. I woke from these aberrations with my face and pillow wet with tears. Sleepcrying.

NIGHT OF THE BIG FIGHT

The rescue joined my brother Billy and me inextricably. As I grew, I'd hear stories of one person saving another's life and how the rescued one was always on the lookout to return the favor, but she also ran the risk of becoming a pest or, worse yet, of living her life in the shadow of her hero. I doggie-paddled through those early years and leaned into my hero, feeling a sense of safety in his presence of which I was unaware.

"Now don't you make your brother carry you." The screen door banged behind my mother's voice. I turned to wave good-bye. She was hazy through the net.

"I won't." Maybe I was four and Billy, thirteen.

We walked hand in hand down the long hill of Glennon Road past many houses that looked alike but for their colors, blue or gray or white. The Vincents' dog ran to the edge of their lawn, barking protectively as we passed, and Billy stood tall. The dog was shaggy black and white except on St. Patrick's Day when his family dyed his white patches green.

Turning into the empty lot near the end of the street, we padded the path cut between weeds by lots of children's feet. I could barely see above those weeds. I loved the way they sounded in the wind, hushing in an almost holy way. The sky was blue, as a May sky should be—Mary's blue, my mother would have said. We were going to

Norm's Store. I didn't know why and didn't care, skipping to keep up with my brother.

The path turned up a little hill and the old oak tree presented itself. I loved that gentlemanly grandfather of a tree. It marked the end of our neighborhood and the beginning of the undeveloped land to the north. It meant that soon we'd be adventuring through a thick of trees, the creek singing beside us. Ahead there'd be the wide open fields that led to Route 155 and the grocery store.

My brother kept a steady pace, but I craned my neck to see if I could see my house. No. I was free and flitted in circles like a buzzing bee. And then—"I'm tiiiiiiired." I stretched the word as I stopped abruptly, leaning against the fat trunk of the old oak.

Billy's brush cut was the same color as the fields. He smiled and I felt like I was seeing his face for the first time ever. He wasn't much for small talk. His eyes crinkled yes, and up I went, up to be the queen carried on top of his strong shoulders.

He was a sensitive boy, nervous, high-strung, who loved music and poetry. I envied his dark blond, wavy hair. When people called him skinny, he'd reply, *I'm not skinny, I'm wiry.*

Billy's gentleness irked my father. Dad couldn't seem to recognize his own exhaustion in getting sober let alone wrangle it. He took it out on everyone, especially his eldest son. Nothing was ever good enough—his grades, his growing hair, his growing silences. Often, there were arguments at our dinner table, the five children and Dad sitting while Mom served and leaned against the kitchen counter. There was not enough room at the table, she said, and she preferred to stand anyway. I practiced my invisibility and at the same time felt cowardly, completely powerless to protect my protector in any way. There were big, mad-dog fights and gnawing, nagging, picking ones, but I don't remember Billy saying one single solitary word, ever.

It was dark outside, a winter night with wind like in a scene from *Dark Shadows*, the show about vampires that I was forbidden to watch because it was sacrilegious, but I did anyway at my friend Dee Korzinski's house.

I must have been about eight.

I sat on the hardwood floor upstairs in my sisters' bedroom, arms tucked around bent legs for safety's sake, and nursed a sinking Sunday night feeling while the radiator blasted hot air. It was the perfect spot to stay warm and to hear my parents' fight echo up the vent.

The door was closed and thank goodness my sisters and I were on the inside. Pat (about nineteen), sat on a chair pulled close to the icy window, which was open a crack, a second-hand fur coat over her shoulders. She smoked cigarettes gingerly while melting red sealing wax to the envelope of a letter she'd just finished. Patty used fountain pens and, if I was lucky, I'd get to stamp the melted wax, creating a regal fleur-de-lis. It tickled my sisters to teach me big words and the Greek alphabet. Mary Ann (about eighteen) studied at her desk. Their transistor radio played a sad-voiced man:

Sittin' here resting my bones
And this loneliness won't leave me alone

A full-length mirror in the shape of a peanut hung on the wall above the radiator vent. I loved my reflection and pretended it was my twin.

I wore a white-flannel, long-sleeved nightgown with red rose-buds, white satin trim, and three pearly buttons at the collar. It was a Christmas tradition to receive pj's or a nightie. The puffed sleeves used to be gathered at the wrists but my mom had cut the elastic because I hated anything tight around my wrists or ankles. She had also run my nightgown through the dryer just before I changed into it, but the cozy feeling had long since grown cold. My feet were sweaty in furry, blue slippers but my hands were icy. I placed one against my mirror-self—icy too.

I practiced my smile and then my puppy dog face, staring deeply into my root beer barrel eyes, like my dad's. My lucky sisters and Billy got Mom's blue eyes, but Danny and I got brown. My hair was a soft brown too, cut short so it wouldn't be trouble to my mother. No time for brushing through snarls with five kids and a house to run. My bangs hung crookedly from a home trim. I had nagged my sisters into fastening three bristly rollers into my bob, one on each side of my head and one on top. They wore huge rollers too. My right ear stuck out a bit from the time I got my head stuck between the railings on Uncle Joe's porch and my dad had to pull hard to get it unstuck. I didn't care, though. It beat what I'd thought he was going to do with the hammer he'd fetched.

"Off with her head," my mother had teased, like the Queen of Hearts from *Alice in Wonderland*.

I was obsessed with decapitation because my paternal grandmother's second cousin, Robert Emmet, the famous Irish patriot and rebel, was hanged, drawn and quartered, and then beheaded. They paraded his noggin about the gallows and proclaimed to the multitudes, "This is the head of a traitor, Robert Emmet."

I was afraid of becoming a traitor.

I was supposed to be brave through centuries of oppression like my ancestors. My great-grandfather, Joseph Connell, was a Nationalist and member of the Irish Republican Brotherhood, a secret oath-bound, fraternal organization dedicated to freeing Ireland. He was a blacksmith and powerful man in Castletown Geoghegan, County Westmeath, second only to the village priest. My dad said Joseph kept a pike hidden beneath the floor of his cottage and always slept with one eye open. I couldn't imagine ever getting to sleep with one eye open—it was hard enough with two closed.

Violence was part of our inheritance.

"You really burn me up," my father's voice boomed up the radiator shaft.

"Aw, go to hell in a handbasket then," my mother roared back.

My sisters smoked and read and turned up the radio.

I looked to my mirror-twin for help, but she shivered in her slippers. *Baby.*

Suddenly, I remembered I wasn't alone. Looking down, there was Shrinking Violet lying belly-up on the floor. I took her soft hand in mine. She was my cloth doll, like Raggedy Ann only better because she was the star of my favorite television cartoon. When she was in trouble, she'd magically shrink and escape. My Shrinking Violet had a big, round head and yellow-yarn hair that I liked to braid. Her purple dress was sewn right onto her body and she had a very flat bottom that stored her audio device. I yanked the little white ring by her neck. A long string pulled taut and she whined, "I'm afraid of noisy boys." All the while, her felt eyelashes blinked up and down, and her sewn lips moved in circles. I hated her weakling voice and frightened face that seemed to worry more when I considered turning her over my knee. I couldn't decide whether to give her a wallop for being a big, fat crybaby or to hug her to me.

Sitting in my sisters' room, I thought about how my mom hadn't spanked me in a long, long time. The last time was a few years before the night of the big fight. We'd been alone in the kitchen.

"I said stop that crying or I'll give you something to cry about."

"I'm not crying. I'm not crying." I gulped and swallowed. I didn't know what I'd done, but I knew Mom was going to hit me because she dragged me by the arm to turn on the radio above the sink to hide her noisy hollers from the neighbors. She got out the metal spatula from the drawer.

If I could have, I would have begged, *I am not a pancake.*

"Turn over."

I tried to pull away.

She pushed me hard to the welcome mat inside the kitchen door, never letting go of my arm. I went limp and let her bend me over. In church, we beseeched Almighty God for mercy. I looked back at her one last time, begging with my face. The spatula was raised high above her head, her teeth bared, the wicked wolf.

She stopped, her hand frozen in mid-air like in a game of freeze tag, staring down the hall.

I followed her gaze to see my daddy in his gray Schaefer Brewery uniform, cap in hand and jacket over his arm. He surprised us, coming in through the front door and bringing a gust of wintry air with him. He looked surprised too and sad to see us so. His face winced and I thought he might cry. I had never seen him cry. My mother released my arm; I ran to him and he picked me up in his big arms. I rested my head on his cold shoulder and held on tight, like a baby monkey.

My mother's voice ringing up the radiator brought me back to the row downstairs. "Wake up the whole neighborhood, why don't you?"

"I oughta skin you alive," Dad hollered and I remembered how he liked to threaten with his huge fist, though I'd never seen him use it—only an open hand to spank my brothers.

"Not if I skin you alive first," shouted Mom. I imagined her face, tomato red.

An even bet.

Then the sound of something smashing ricocheted around the radiator, maybe a cup or saucer thrown and shattered against the wall.

Then silence.

"Come away from there, Kitten." Mary Ann led me to her desk. The bristly rollers would style her hair like Laura Petrie's from *The Dick Van Dyke Show*. She knew how much I loved to sit at that desk, surrounded by the halo of her study lamp. She handed me a photo album with a red burlap cover. Inside were boring postcards of ancient city buildings from her German pen pal. I flipped page after page to find the one different from the rest, an Easter card of Peter Rabbit. He looked guilty as an angry-faced Mother Rabbit pulled his long ear. On the ground in front of him was a huge, elaborately painted Easter egg, broken in two. I knew that boy bunny had done it.

Suddenly, I worried. Where were my brothers?

Just then, the door to my sisters' room burst open and the boys wrestled in.

"Coast is clear, time for bed, Kathy," Billy announced while holding Danny in a headlock and tickling him unmercifully. Dan wore a German helmet, the souvenir Dad had brought home from the war.

"Daddy's driving away, up the hill now." Patty snubbed out a cigarette, turning from the window.

"Uncle, uncle!" Danny begged.

The boys must have been across the hall in Billy's room during our parents' fight.

Billy released Danny from the wrestling hold and Danny jumped around, a monkey high on Mallo Cups, the yellow wrapper still clenched in his paw. He wore brown polyester pajama pants and a brown, white, and orange striped long-sleeved pajama top.

"Time to go to bed, Baby-Kathy, time for your bottle and blanky," Dan taunted.

Strangers thought we were twins even though he was two years older, even though I was skinny and he was husky. That's what my mom called it, husky. Dad would sing at dinner, "Danny is a pelican. His beak holds more than his belly can."

"I'll take them down," Patty offered.

Next thing I remember, I was lying in my twin bed in the first-floor room I shared with Danny, next to the kitchen. Most nights it was prime realty because we could easily raid the kitchen on tiptoe if our parents were watching television in the living room or sleeping in their bedroom, both at the other end of the hall. But on a night like this, I longed for upstairs.

Dan fell asleep quickly in spite of the big fight and the candy. He snored softly from across the room.

My oldest sister sat on the edge of my bed, facing me, those rollers like fat caterpillars crawling her skull.

"Please take mine out. I can't sleep with them."

And she removed my beauty treatment.

"How do I look?"

Pondering, "Handsome."

A boy was the last thing I wanted to look like.

Patty was beautiful with long, dark hair against fair skin and Paul Newman eyes. She was a wonderful artist who taught me to draw and paint. I imagined we were Meg and Amy in *Little Women*, bound together as the oldest and youngest.

Patty had penciled my portrait when I was four, a profile. It was pensive, everybody joked, because even though I watched *The Jetsons* while she drew, my expression was furrowed, my lower lip pouted. I hated when George got stuck on a moving sidewalk and how no one heard him when he yelped for help. I knew it was supposed to be funny; everyone else laughed.

I squeezed my sister's hand, begging her not to go.

I said the prayer to my guardian angel and offered my sleeplessness and my handsomeness up for the poor souls in purgatory.

"Will you sing 'More' to me?"

And she did.

My life will be in your keeping, waking, sleeping, laughing, weeping,
Longer than always is a long, long time, but far beyond forever you'll be mine.

Then she sang about a cruel war raging, a boy named Johnny who had to fight, and his sweetheart who pleaded to tie up her hair, wear men's clothing, and pretend to be his comrade.

Won't you let me go with you?
No, my love, no.

I wished I could take my sister into sleep with me. By this time, Patty had entertained me enough and hinted at leaving.

"Why can't I sleep upstairs with you and Mary Ann? I implore you!" We both smiled at my use of the new vocabulary word.

"No room," she'd whisper.

Finally, we played our favorite bedtime game where Patty hummed "The Funeral March" by Chopin while ever-so-slowly pulling the blankets up over my face like a dead little girl being laid to rest. As she approached the end of the musical phrase and once my head was completely covered, she popped the covers off: "Boo!"

We found the ritual hysterical and broke into peals of hushed laughter.

Eventually, Patricia had to leave me and I felt my body grow cold—a real, live, dead girl.

I lay there and time passed.

I stared hard through the dark at Danny, willing him awake, but he snored away.

The door was open and light from the television flashed down the hall. I heard *Mission Impossible* voices so it must have been after ten o'clock. They were mixed in a jumble with the scary voices inside my head, speaking of going to hell in a handbasket after being skinned alive. The wind picked up and rattled both windows in our corner room. I thought again about *Dark Shadows* and how I'd deceived my mother by watching it at the Korzinskis' and how maybe God was punishing me now with sleeplessness. I said an Act of Contrition.

O my God, I am heartily sorry for having offended Thee,
and I detest all my sins, because I dread the loss of heaven,
and the pains of hell; but most of all because they offend Thee, my God,
Who are all good and deserving of all my love.
I firmly resolve, with the help of Thy grace,
to confess my sins, to do penance,
and to amend my life. Amen.

I had to pee but held it, because if I stepped off the edge of the bed, the devil might drag me under.

Slivers of light from the moon slipped through the window blinds. Those blinds looked like bones in an X-ray from a scene in *Dr. Kildare*, which my mother didn't care for because it was a kind of soap opera, but Colleen O'Keefe—my other neighborhood friend—her mother did. Was it a sin to watch a show your mother didn't like, even if it was not a sacrilegious show but only a kind of soap opera?

I murmured another Act of Contrition. Better safe than sorry.

Think happy thoughts, my mom counseled me once when I'd asked her advice on falling asleep.

I imagined Bing Crosby and Rosemary Clooney in *White Christmas*.

If you're worried and you can't sleep
Just count your blessings instead of sheep.

My sheets were flowered and my pillowcase striped and I loved flowers and stripes. I hugged my candy blanket in appreciation, spread over me on this bitter night. Grandma Frazier had won it at a fair. It had crocheted patches of color against black, like candies on a counter, perfect for playing store.

I listed more blessings:

Vacations in Camp Billy two weeks every summer with the whole family in the Thousand Islands and walks to the candy store for King Cones.

My big Christmas present, a red wheelie bike with streamers like Eddie Munster's.

The smell of Patricia's makeup bag and my mom's Chanel No 5.

Dashing to the kitchen upon waking to beat Danny to the creamy, sugary sip of coffee Dad left in the bottom of his cup for us.

Cuddling Mom when she'd take a break from reading her newspapers.

Mommy's macaroni and cheese with tomatoes. Beef stew. Browned pork chops.

Sitting by the radiator eating boiled potatoes with lots of butter and salt and pepper after coming in from sledding the other day.

I thought about the night before the night of the big fight, of dancing with my father to *The Lawrence Welk Show*, my legs dangling as we bounced around the living room. He was so handsome in his fancy suit, and Mom was beautiful with her fox stole with the real fox face around her coat collar, ready for their meeting-date. "Remember," she'd whispered to me, "if the neighbors ask, we've gone to a *union* meeting." Really they were off to be with his sober friends. She kissed my cheek, leaving behind a perfect, red lip-print that I admired when Dad and I lingered at the mirror that hung above the couch.

Danny and I had leaned against the storm door, fogging it with our breath and drawing funny faces on the glass as our parents drove away, up Glennon Road and out of sight. We chanted, "Going, going, going, going, going, going, going, going, going, going, going, going, going, going, *gone!*"

It seemed so long ago, the night of the meeting-date, and I sang softly, in an effort to bring it back, the encore song from *The Lawrence Welk Show*.

Goodnight, sleep tight, and pleasant dreams to you
Here's a wish and a prayer that every dream comes true.

I was grateful for our warm house and said another prayer, this time for the poor children of Africa even though I was pretty sure they were suffering from heat exhaustion and not hypothermia. I felt a sinking feeling that they were pagans, which wasn't their fault but if we didn't support our missionaries and christen the African babies, soon they'd all land in Limbo like Sister Mary Thomas said.

I thought about Sister Mary Thomas's mustache and heavy hand with the ruler, and I wondered if she was really a man pretending to be a nun. I wished the pretty actress in *The Flying Nun* was my teacher and that Limbo did not exist. It seemed so unfair, like going to sleep. I wondered if going to Limbo was as bad or worse than going to sleep.

I hated Sunday nights and the sickening feeling of the school week stretched out before me, slow torture.

I thought about what I called torture movies. I was allowed to watch them if they were classics, by which I figured Mom meant black and white. There was *The Man in the Iron Mask*, in which a prince suffered with his face shut up tight, nearly strangling himself with his own beard because his jealous brother, the king, had locked him away in a dungeon.

The Man in the Iron Mask was only a made-up torture movie, I told myself, not real life. Even though Mary Ann, who loved all things historical, said it was based on the true story of a French guy imprisoned by King Louis the XIV.

I decided that going to sleep was like being shut up in a metal mask.

I knew I'd derailed far from the happy-thought track.

My hands clenched Brownie, my well-worn, dark-chocolate-brown teddy bear. I was grateful for Brownie and that I could hear our car pull up, meaning my father had come home from wherever he'd gone.

I loved my daddy. He was the only father in the neighborhood who'd pile a gang of us kids into his car on summer nights and buy us ice cream cones near the airport so we could watch the planes fly over our heads to land.

I lay very still and searched my heart for more blessings, but there was a pulsing in my ears that drove me crazy. I didn't move. I couldn't. I felt paralyzed. The pulsing spoke to me, "I am going to skin you alive . . ." It echoed round my head, a fever voice, only my forehead was cool.

I didn't know what to believe, the memory of my father's embrace or the memory of his fighting voice ringing first up the radiator and then around my worrywart head. The garage door opened and I counted fifteen Mississippis as he parked the car and closed the garage door. Then the kitchen door opened and I heard him stomping snow off his boots.

I pretended to sleep.

Daddy moved past my door and I heard my parents' bedroom door close. The television continued blaring *Mission Impossible* as if nothing had happened. Time passed. Against my might, and stiff arms and legs, sleep began to overtake me. In the moment of letting go, I heard Danny from across the room, crying in his dream or maybe he'd been awake for awhile.

"Are you all right?"

"I'm fine. Go back to sleep," he whispered.

More time passed and I noticed someone had turned off the TV. I began to doze until Danny's voice broke through the silence, "Kathy, if you had a choice, would you rather die by getting your head chopped off, or like Sister Martin's cousin who was caught in a fire and wrapped a rug around himself crawling 'cross the burning room on his belly, only the rug had rubber on the bottom side and melted together making a trap so he couldn't move and burned slowly alive?"

"Head chopped off."

"Me too. Good night."

More time passed, though I couldn't say how much, and I was drifting again through the wide expanse between awake and asleep when I heard Danny's voice from far away.

"Kathy...would you pick up my head? It just rooooooooooooooolled on the floor."

I heard a loud, long scream, a torture movie scream. It was me screaming and I couldn't stop. It was no nightmare. It was real, and Danny hooted from across the room.

My mother boomed down the corridor, grabbing the yardstick from the hall closet outside our bedroom. Danny burrowed under the covers. He'd dragged his pillow with him and I knew he was padding his bottom. At first my brother laughed because he was tricking her, but Mommy dragged him out and beat him with that wooden stick anyway.

"I told you not to tease your sister, you . . . "

And then to me, "Are you happy now? Are you satisfied?"

I covered my ears and shrunk myself, wishing I could be more like Shrinking Violet in her cartoon show when she'd disappear for safety's sake. I pretended invisibility beneath the candy blanket. I couldn't save Danny from my mother any more than I could save Billy from my father. I wasn't brave like Robert Emmet. I was a coward. I was a traitor.

FIRST SLEEPWALK

The first time I sleepwalked was the summer of 1970. I was ten. Danny had been moved upstairs to Billy's room. Patty and Mary Ann, twenty-one and twenty respectively, continued to share the other second floor bedroom. The three oldest were, each in their own way, beginning to separate from the family and I dreaded the idea of losing them.

As the sole kid on the first floor with my siblings camped in pairs above me, I felt left out. At bedtime, I was dismissed with a kiss and a "pleasant dreams," which I believed *must* be returned, spoken by all family members, present and accounted for, or else something terrible would befall us in the dark. From the beginning, I was waiting, waiting for that catastrophe. I was sent to bed earliest but fought against sleep 'til the bitter end. I didn't want to miss anything, good or bad.

It was a humid night and hardly anybody had air-conditioning yet. Crickets chirped through the open windows; blinds were up and curtains pulled back to let in the still air. I pulled the sheet over my head despite the heat. I hated that there was only the flimsy screen between the night and me. I'd added Peeping Toms to my list of fears.

Around this time a creeper had been seen in our neighborhood, a two-street community in a working-class suburb. One night, the police were called because Patty had been frightened coming home from a date. As the littlest, and as a part of *being so quiet you wouldn't even know I was there*, I'd gathered enough information to thoroughly scare myself.

Sometimes teenagers from the larger, newer, and therefore more dangerous neighborhood behind ours, cut through our street to get to the liquor store in the strip mall on Route 9 or to party in the fields north of our development. I was jealous of their freshly built, split-level ranch houses on streets named Aurora or Lakewood, and I imagined them living groovy *Brady Bunch* lives.

Raucous laughter blasted in waves as they passed our house that night and I feared their public school reputations. I felt isolated even if my family was a few rooms away watching *NBC Saturday Night at the Movies*.

I don't know how much time passed while I lay there parsing every sound.

The room moved in circles between awake and asleep. I felt everything spinning. Instinctively, I knew that I could keep it spinning simply by concentrating on the spinning.

Finally I fell away.

I don't know how long I slept before I stirred.

They said I walked as though without a care down the hall toward the light of the TV. I stood perfectly still in the doorway that led to the living room and stared straight ahead, eyes wide open—a mannequin.

My mother glanced up first. She was sitting in the green recliner. "Kathy," she questioned, almost as if she didn't recognize me, "what are you doing up?"

I didn't answer. I gazed straight ahead, blinking. My older brothers and sisters laughed.

"She's not herself," someone said.

"She's sleepwalking," Billy realized.

"Go back to bed, honey. It's late." They were calm, bemused.

I turned away, a little smile on my face, an obedient budding somnambulist, and walked back to bed unattended, gliding almost ghostly, as though above the floor.

In the morning, eating toast at the kitchen table, I remembered nothing.

Nothing at all.

My siblings laughed as they told me what happened.

I felt like I had played a trick on them. *I am so powerful. I can move in my sleep and I don't even know it.* But then I thought about my mom tearing through the house in the middle of the night. I worried that it would happen to me again. Maybe next time it wouldn't be so funny. I felt sick and stopped eating breakfast.

Did some part of me remember my mother's voice, distant as though through a fever, "Kathy? What are you doing up?"

I wanted to remember. I wanted to.

Sleepwalking. I could leave my body and become a spirit, *Casper the Friendly Ghost*, even though I let my body tag along.

"You were so funny," someone teased, "like Norton in the *Honeymooners*, sleepwalking while looking for his long lost dog, Lulu. Only his eyes were shut and yours were wide open and glazed over."

"Did you have a nightcap, Kathy?" somebody joked.

"Like your soul had been snatched," Billy added, "like in *Night Gallery*."

"Don't say that," snapped my mother.

But everyone else laughed and I laughed too.

We kids couldn't possibly fathom the depth of Mom's fear based on her own experience.

For a few years, I sleepwalked as though in a trance, as though hypnotized by a magician. Episodes were eerie but without the added panic of violence and night terrors. When I was twelve, that would all change.

ST. DYMPHNA'S DAY

My mom took the call late afternoon on May 15, 1972, the Monday after Mother's Day. How weighty our black rotary phone must have been, the news adding a considerable load. Billy had been serving in the army, stationed in Germany. He'd enlisted after hearing a rumor that it lessened your chances of being sent to Vietnam and his draft number was coming up anyway.

I wasn't home when we got word. After school, I'd gone directly to hang out with my best friend and neighbor, Colleen O'Keefe, who lived across the street. Before I'd left for school, there'd been twinges in my right ear. By the time I returned from Colleen's, it ached. I got chronic ear infections and dreaded the piercing pain that was on its way.

The house was deserted except for the sound of weeping coming up from the basement. I opened the door and descended the stairs nervously.

We kids were forever turning off the lights on each other down there and jumping out from behind stacked boxes. The stairs had no backs to them, just splintering planks of wood. I was always afraid I would slip between them into the darkness, a sacrifice to the bogeyman.

My mother's back was to me as she ironed under the solitary bare bulb. Her shoulders shook from crying. Dull light bled through the few small windows where the walls met the ceiling. The one above the washer and dryer framed the rusty, overturned wheelbarrow on our backyard lawn. Mom loved to keep our windows sparkling but those that lined the cellar were webbed in dirt.

Despite the chill, she wore a muumuu over a man's T-shirt. She was going through the change of life and flushed so hot sometimes she'd have to stop whatever she was doing and sit, grabbing a newspaper for a fan. Her ankles ballooned over gray Hush Puppies.

My mother was pressing a pair of Billy's pajamas. I'd never seen her iron nightclothes before. She hadn't heard me tiptoe down the stairs and suddenly tipped the iron upright to rest on the board. She placed my brother's pajama top over her shoulder and patted it, like you would to soothe a baby, caught her breath between sobs, and sang the lullaby she'd made up for us kids.

Once I had a baby, a baby, a baby,
Once I had a baby, an old tomato patch
Billy is that baby, that baby, that baby,
Billy is that baby, that old tomato patch.

"Damn it," she said, a quiet apology for her tears that had fallen onto her work. "I'm gonna have to wash you again."

Mom covered her face with the flannel top and her whole body shook violently. I had no idea what to do. I cleared my throat and she turned, lowering the shirt. Her blue eyes were made even more cadet blue from crying and I thought, *She must have been a beautiful girl.*

"Kathy." She motioned me closer and I tentatively edged toward her. When I stepped within arm's reach, she hugged me to her suddenly, ferociously.

"What's wrong? What is it, Ma?"

Then she sort of pushed me away and I stood frozen to the spot where I landed.

"Pass me those sheets."

She threw the tear-stained pj's into the dirty laundry basket on the floor and began pressing sheets with a heavy hand. "He was a beautiful child, a head full of golden ringlets. He'd play for hours while I sat and read the papers, toy soldiers climbing up my shoes for hills. . . . Look at that."

She paused to show me the flaming red palm of her ironing hand.

"I don't have to grip it so hard. Remember to let the iron do its work, Kathy. I should know better . . . I should have known better. . . ." I somehow knew she wasn't talking about her task at hand. Pulling tissues from her pocket, she dabbed her puffed face. "I'll never forgive that quack, the way he bruised Billy's perfect head with those damn forceps."

"What's wrong with Billy?"

"I forgot. You weren't here."

"Is he all right?"

She dropped her head into the crook of her arm and whispered, "He's more than a stone's throw from all right, Kathy." My heart dropped to my stomach. I took a giant step back and pressed against the whirring washer as it entered its spin cycle. She looked at me then and spoke calmly, "Your brother suffered a nervous breakdown. The army's going to fly him to the states just as soon as he's able. Then Daddy and Danny and you and I will drive down to the hospital in Pennsylvania to see him."

I guessed the chronic ear infections had damaged my hearing because I had no idea what she was saying but I was afraid to press her. She was a wild card, my mother, and could fly from maudlin to furious before I could even figure out what had set her off.

Still I had to know, "What . . . happened?"

She looked away again and leaned into her work with her full weight. When she answered, she spoke slowly, "Your brother attempted suicide."

As torturous as it was to the both of us, I still didn't understand, "What do you mean?"

She paused for a long time, not bothering to lift the iron from the sheet even when I worried it might scorch. Her voice ached with the truth. "He cut his wrists as if to take his life."

My head pounded worse than ever. Something was stuck in there and begging, *Uncle, Uncle*. I turned away and pressed my bad ear on a stack of neatly folded towels, still warm from the dryer. My mother's breath ran away from her in grunts and I remembered a mommy bear on *Discovery* who couldn't free her cub from a trap. Then the basement was still except for the sounds of the machines.

After a while, there was the hiss of the iron at work again. Mommy whispered, "He jumped out of a second-story window when he was thirteen. I never told you that, did I, Kathy? He was trying to get away from your father . . . one of his goddamn fits of rage." *Sisssssssssssssss*, the iron continued. "I never . . . should have married the son of a bitch . . . I should have stayed in the navy."

I stared down at my new Keds and worried, would I have been born? I felt bad for thinking about myself at a time like this.

"Do you know what else today is?"

I turned to face my mother and shook my head no.

"It's St. Dymphna's Feast Day. St. Dymphna, patron saint of the mentally ill. Maybe . . . it isn't entirely my fault," and she broke down into another series of heartbreaking sobs.

I felt glued to the basement floor, a cartoon character—unable to comfort my mother. Besides, if I touched her she might break into a million pieces.

It seemed I would never fall asleep that night, as the storm that had threatened all day turned into a relentless downpour. There were no streetlights in our little neighborhood and no reflection from the television this evening. Quiet, except for the rain, and whispers, and tears from my parents' room down the hall.

I was willing to bet that my father would be up all night, what with his worry gene and all. Before Billy had moved out of our house, he'd been picked on more and more for his unruly long hair, his poor grades at community college, his hippie friends. My father had lost control over his son. It culminated in a frantic dance between them in our kitchen one night. My dad grabbed at my brother's shirt sleeves and Billy backed away in a circle until my father grasped the material and shoved it up above his elbow, screaming, "What's that, what's that, what are those marks?" I had no idea what the needle scars on the inside of my brother's arm meant, but he moved out soon after.

On the night of the day of the bad news, I grabbed the flashlight that I kept tucked in Flower's sewn embrace. She was a bunny, one of a dozen stuffed animals that covered the crack between my bed and the wall, my guards against the underworld. Using my covers for a tent, I leafed through my *Little Book of Saints* and found the holy card my mother had given me of St. Dymphna, remembering her words as she'd handed it to me, *You know, Kathy, she's patron saint of sleepwalkers, too.*

The martyred Irish princess looked especially saintly in my flashlight's halo and I turned over the card to read her prayer.

O God, we humbly beseech You through Your servant, St Dymphna, who sealed with her blood the love she bore You, to grant relief to those who suffer from mental afflictions and nervous disorders, especially, (_____). Amen.

I filled in the blank with Billy's name.

Dymphna lived during the seventh century. Her mom died when she was fifteen and her dad, a pagan king, grew mentally ill with grief. When he couldn't find a new wife who resembled his first, he became obsessed with marrying his daughter. She ran away but was caught in Belgium, where her father beheaded her. Hundreds of years later, in Gheel, on the site of her decapitation, some sick and suffering medieval souls, wandering and homeless, fell asleep and woke up free from mental illness.

My ear continued to ache and I longed for a heating pad but I hadn't told my mother. I hated the eardrops that ran inside my head and preferred to offer my agony up for the sake of my brother. I tucked St. Dymphna's holy card under my pillow and lay on my side, turning my bad ear toward the image. I thought about Billy's face underwater when he'd rescued me and how I was unable to save him now. I couldn't bear thinking about him across the great Atlantic Ocean, waves and waves away.

A long time passed. Still no sleep.

I removed my brown scapular from around the bedpost and blew off the dust, repentant for letting it hang unattended. There were two squares of felt attached to brown cord, to be worn together. One held the image of the most Holy Virgin Mary and the other, her promise, "Whosoever dies wearing this scapular shall not suffer eternal fire."

Sister Mary Gerard, my seventh-grade teacher, had lectured that suicide was a mortal sin. Mortal. To burn in unimaginable torment for eternity. I worried if Billy had his scapular across the sea. Maybe if I'd kept my promise to wear Mary's scapular always, my brother would not have done what he'd done. I placed it around my neck, despite my fear of it tangling and choking me to death in my sleep. I vowed to wear it always and forever, truly this time. I begged Our Lady to bring him home safe and sound.

Lying in bed on the night of the day of the bad news, I began to cry. It was ridiculous for me to imagine that my prayers could help. Deep down inside, I knew I was the opposite of saintly. I was a liar. And one of my falsehoods had hurt Billy and hurt him badly.

The year before, I'd gone with some older kids to Saratoga Performing Arts Center to hear Chicago. We'd sat on a blanket on the lawn. Before the show began, a nearby radio blasted Country Joe and the Fish's antiwar song, "The Fish Cheer & I Feel Like I'm Fixing to Die Rag." It began:

Gimme an F! (and the crowd screamed F)

Gimme an I! (but the crowd screamed U)

Gimme an S! (but the crowd screamed C)

Gimme an H! (but the crowd screamed K)

I understood that the big kids despised the Vietnam War and that *fuck* was a forbidden, angry word, but I was unaware of the sexual meaning. Some days later, I found myself alone and standing in the hallway of the first floor of our house with a pen in my hand. I felt possessed. Someone was moving my body while my mind drifted away. Was I sleepwalking? Had I been napping? But my episodes were only at night. I had no idea what I was mad about, but I was writing the word *fuck* on our closed basement door. I got through writing the F and U, about ten inches tall, when I realized the permanence of my prank since the pen had actually scratched the letters into the wood. I crossed them out as though that would make it better.

But the worst part, the absolute shameful part, was when my parents accused Billy of the vandalism. I cowardly held my tongue and let him take the blame. His voice plaintively denied the crime, but I'd been too afraid of what the punishment might be to come clean.

God, I felt guilty about that as I lay, stuck in bed, incapable of soothing anyone, ever. Clearly, I was a sinful girl and I'd been stupid to aspire to sainthood. I cried for my brother and the wrong I had done him. I lost all track of time lying there self-flagellating. My parents' whispers and tears continued. With my good ear, I listened to the rain shake the windows as if trying to bring the whole house back to its senses. I pressed my bad ear into the pillow. I touched St. Dymphna's card to be sure it was still there.

Eventually, I must have fallen asleep.

The next day, I was up before dawn and overheard my parents' voices through their bedroom door, which had been left opened a bit. I couldn't resist leaning close to spy, one of my favorite Invisible Girl games. That's how I found out what my mother and I had done on the night of the bad news.

My dad had awoken in the middle of the night and couldn't get back to sleep. He whispered the Five Sorrowful Mysteries of the Rosary, quietly so as not to wake his wife. He'd been begging mercy for his son when my mother called out from deep inside her slumber, "My boy, my boy," and jumped up to save my brother from every parent's worst nightmare. She ran top speed into the hall but her golden-haired boy was nowhere to be found.

At that same moment, I hollered and also dashed into the hallway, colliding with Mom, crashing full force as we each flailed about, lost in the thick of our *very, very bad nightmares.*

Dad separated us and got us back to our beds. He said that afterward we each fell into a heavy sleep, as is common on the heels of an episode—like an epileptic kid he grew up with, he noticed. As if the fit had taken everything out of us, and it was like a fit of sorts, wasn't it?

I remembered nothing.

After eavesdropping, I slumped to the kitchen, filled a hot water bottle, and went to my room to rest. I was freaked out about running through our hallway while sound asleep. I was just like my mother. With my bad ear pressed to the warmth, I thought for a long time about the scene my dad had described. His voice had reminded me of Rod Serling's when, at the top of each *Night Gallery* episode, he introduced the gruesome tale that followed. It horrified me, hearing my father talk that way. I'd been caught in a scene from that creepy television show, possessed, and my mother too, and I thought of my brother—worst of all—far across the dangerous sea.

It was too awful to hold in my mind, so I unpacked my memory of the previous night, weighing each bedtime thought, turning them over one by one in my little girl hands. I grasped on how I'd let Billy take the blame for my vandalism of the basement door. Surely that was the reason God had punished me with the *very, very bad nightmare.*

My throat was sore, as though I had hollered long and hard like Dad said, but wouldn't it have woken me? And what about my siblings upstairs? Had it woken them? Maybe they'd stopped running to help at every holler in the middle of the night.

I was Dr. Jekyll and Mr. Hyde, an A student and phony holy girl by day but at night I became my real self, a monster. I closed my eyes and pressed my mind to recall any detail of my walking night-mare. Was I imagining it or did part of me remember the mad dance of flailing arms with my mother in our darkened hall? A feeling of impending doom came back to me and a sense of running from whomever, whatever was coming to get me. Or maybe I was just making that up. Lying in bed, longing for the respite of an afternoon nap, the incident escalated in my mind, ending in my secret fear of falling down the cellar stairs, slipping through the wooden planks to my death. Thank goodness the basement door had been closed, or had it? I couldn't ask without hinting that I knew about the incident. Better to just play along and hope it wouldn't happen again. I almost laughed aloud at my stupid self. I was ridiculous to think things would get anything but worse.

ONE FLEW OVER THE CUCKOO'S NEST

After my brother took ill, when I sleepwalked it was usually coupled with panic. It was the intensity of my nocturnal wandering, regardless of the frequency, the total loss of control that frightened me the most during early adolescence.

Billy was flown from Germany to Fort Dix Air Force Base in New Jersey, where he stayed for a few days before being admitted to the locked psychiatric ward of the Valley Forge Veterans Administration Hospital in Pennsylvania. Patricia and Mary Ann stayed home, due to school and work, but Mom, Dad, Danny, and I visited him the first chance we could.

We went straight to the hospital when we got there. Dad turned off the engine and leaned his head against the steering wheel. Mom applied blood-red lipstick, perfectly, in the rear view mirror that she'd turned toward the passenger's seat. Danny and I stared. We were entranced by her business-as-usual attitude.

"We've got to show Billy that everything is going to be okay, back to normal, that this was just a one-time incident."

Silence.

She removed tissue from the sleeve of her sweater and pressed it between her lips and then she dabbed the clean part against the corners of her eyes to wipe away the tears.

"Reach in the glove compartment, will ya, Kate, and hand me the directions on where we're supposed to go?"

I rested my head against the closed window and looked at the maze of two-story buildings constructed of red brick. How would we ever find my brother?

"Darn, I forgot about this!"

Mom had found the Mass card she'd ordered from the Carmelite Friars of Our Lady of Mount Carmel Monastery, in Middletown, New York. While Dad read about where visitors were supposed to check in, Mom filled out Billy's gift. It was a holy greeting card. For just a few dollars, Billy would be remembered in the Masses, prayers, and good works of the Friars for as long as their graces were needed.

"Their prayers will make short order of this mess." She flicked her pen disdainfully toward the institution.

No one answered but we all nodded our heads. It reminded me of those dolls people stick in their back car windows that bob their noggins whenever the vehicle stops or starts.

Once inside, an attendant named Wilber showed us to the wing that housed those who suffered from mental illness. Wilber was young and built like a fortress, taller even than my father's six foot, three inches.

Sunshine flooded the windowed network of corridors. Walking along, I felt strange, very strange. I was there with my family, but I wasn't there. I wanted to see Billy but was terrified too. I thought about the day we heard the bad news, and even though I knew it wasn't realistic, I wished for what life would have been like if my mother had never answered the phone. Maybe this was a bad dream, the kind where I could not escape whoever was coming to get me.

"We're almost there," Wilbur said.

But the closer we came to our destination, the more I felt myself disappear.

We turned a corner, and a door different from the rest waited for us. It was metal with a barred window—the locked door that separated the psychiatric ward. Wilber took a ring of keys from a long chain attached to his belt. He unlocked the door and Danny's chest heaved as though he might sob. Daddy put an arm around him and Mommy reached for my hand. If it weren't for that, I might have floated away completely.

Inside, we sat in a kind of waiting area on orange plastic chairs across from a big window that looked into the nurses' station, but we could not see into the ward. Wilber said someone would be with us soon. He shook my father's hand and left us there. This was where visitors showed identification and were cleared. Opposite the door we'd just entered was another locked door, a twin to the first. I heard noise, lots of noise, from behind the door that lead to the patients, but I couldn't tell what was happening in there. We were in purgatory, stuck between freedom and torture.

A nurse with pursed lips, a starched white cap, and a perfectly white dress called my parents over to a hole in the window. I heard them talking but couldn't comprehend what they were saying, as though English were a foreign language. She nodded sympathetically then disappeared. A buzzer sounded, the second door swung open, and the nurse met us.

She welcomed us into the ward's recreation room where the air hung heavy with piss and cigarette smoke and ammonia. A ping-pong table sat deserted with its net slumping. A TV blared in one corner and a few men in pajamas and robes sat, hypnotized by the show. Others were having conversations with the actors. One patient with greasy hair and a cigarette sat alone babbling on, nonstop, about something scary. He repulsed me and even though I knew it was rude, I had to stare. Everywhere was the same man—only older, younger, fatter, dry, smelly, praying, screaming, pacing, crying, laughing, staring, drooling. Two were dancing cheek to cheek, imitating who I guessed were Fred Astaire and Ginger Rogers waltzing, a swirl of white feathers and black tails, on the set. Most of the patients ignored us, but a few glanced at me as we passed and I felt my face blush red, ashamed for having stared.

The nurse brought us to the visitors' room but there were no other visitors. Barred windows lined one wall. Jail. The sun that glared from the outside world caused lines of shadows to fall across the black and white linoleum floor. Orange tables and couches scattered the room. We sat around a round table and we waited for what seemed like forever.

Wilber returned with the same nurse who had greeted us. She escorted my brother by the elbow. He wouldn't have moved if she hadn't sort of dragged him along. Wilber took over the dragging part and the lady nurse left the room.

Billy didn't seem to recognize us as he shuffled our way.

My mother could not contain herself. She cried and my father took her hand in his and squeezed it hard and steady until she stopped.

Wilber deposited Billy in a chair at our table then went to stand guard, still in the room but just inside the door to give us some privacy. Each of us got up—smiling, smiling, smiling as we gave him hugs. I thought, do they ever wash his hair or give him a bath in this place? Even his green paper slippers made his feet look sickly. His eyes stared blankly. His flannel pajamas and green hospital robe hung loosely on his frame. I thought about how as a kid he used to say, "I'm not skinny, I'm wiry." Now he'd lost all muscle. His youth, his very will to live, seemed to have been drained out of him. I didn't know by whom but vowed then and there to find out. I'd kill the bastard.

He had been diagnosed paranoid schizophrenic and manic depressive, and was definitely down today. He lifted a frail hand as though it weighed a hundred pounds and wiped drool from his chin. His fingers shook like an old man's and were stained orange brown from cigarettes that he forgot he was holding until the near burn of their embers jolted him out of his stupor. Noticing the ashtray in front of him, he removed a pack of unfiltered Lucky Strikes from his pajama top pocket. We all watched, hypnotized by his slow motion moves. He waved the cigarette in the air and mumbled a joke about "you are what you eat," meaning "lucky," I guessed, although none of us cracked a smile. He called out to Wilber for a light. The young attendant complied, almost like a friend to Billy. I didn't understand why my brother was not allowed matches or a lighter. His wrists were still bandaged with gauze where they were healing. His hospital identification band hung loosely there and read WILLIAM E. FRAZIER, but this was not my before brother. What had they done with the boy who had carried me on his shoulders as we'd crossed the fields to Norm's grocery to buy milk for Mom? My stomach hurt, like a sucker punch perfectly placed.

He rocked slowly, as though he was his own baby trying to calm himself, but we pretended not to notice. If he was any calmer, he would have collapsed to the floor.

"I have . . . something . . . for you." He spoke out of one side of his mouth and his cigarette dangled precariously from the other. He reached into his bathrobe pocket and, what seemed like a half hour later, pulled out some yellow, loose-leaf papers and unfolded them.

He snubbed out his smoke in the ashtray as he spoke, "I wrote it . . . when Wilber let me . . . use his pen. Supervised penmanship . . . supervised penmanship," and he sort of grunted a laugh. "These are just a few things . . . they say. I can't . . . get it all down, just a . . . few . . . lines when I'm . . . lucky. Ohhhh, lucky . . . I'm so . . . lucky . . . right, guys?"

Wilber had been leaning against the wall, cleaning his fingernails with a toothpick but he came to attention as Billy delivered his slurred speech. He approached the table quietly and stood behind my brother.

"Billy's been writing some poetry," Wilber said, not unkindly.

"Oh, nooooooooooooooooooooo . . . Man upstairs is the poet . . . I'm just the . . . scribe." The opened papers trembled in his hands and he steadied them by resting them on the table. He closed his eyes for a long time. He had fallen asleep—or maybe the drugs had knocked him out. A string of drool slipped from his mouth and dribbled onto his work.

"Billy," Daddy said as he tenderly placed his big mitt of a hand on his son's delicate one. My brother startled awake and jerked away from Dad's touch. He noticed the spittle pooling on his papers and used his bathrobe sleeve to wipe it away. Dark shame fell across his face, followed by a painful pause. Then, with what felt like a herculean effort, he gathered up his papers and crumpled them. He tried to rip them up but was too weak.

"Easy now, Buddy, easy," Wilber whispered as to a nervous horse and he patted my brother's shoulder. Billy folded his arms on the table, dropped his head like a little, little kid, and sobbed, breaking our hearts.

"I think visiting time's up." The burly attendant lifted my brother from under the arms and practically carried him away. Billy did not at all resist. In fact, his body relaxed, grateful for the young attendant's calm resolve.

Between her own sobs, Mom said she would bring him home soon. Just as soon as the doctors gave the word.

Wilber answered in a voice full of determination, "Billy's much better now, really."

Mom repeated, "Billy's much better now, really."

Well, we could all see that.

Later that night, at the Holiday Inn, Dad discovered the Mass card in his coat pocket and the fact that he'd forgotten to give it to Billy threw Mom into a tantrum.

"That really burns me up," she kept repeating, and I imagined her consumed in flames as she paced the tiny, tan room. When she calmed down enough to sit on one of the beds and watch *All in the Family* with us, she *stewed*, my father said, and her angry face did resemble a stewed tomato.

I couldn't fall asleep. Mom was my bed partner. Dad and Danny shared the other double. I missed my night-light. I'd forgotten my stuffed animals. Even Dad fell asleep before me. My mother's heavy body was a boulder on the bed. I kept rolling toward her. I hated sleeping next to anybody and clung to the edge of the mattress, nearly falling to the dirty rug. Our room was on the second floor. I was closest to the window and jumped every time a car door closed in the parking lot. What stranger passed below?

I knew I had to close my eyes to fall asleep, but every time I did I saw Billy's face twisted in pain in the moment before he broke into sobs at the hospital—or underwater, the time he saved me from drowning at Aunt Kathleen's lake.

"How does Billy sleep at the hospital?" I asked aloud but no one answered. That's how I knew I was the only one left keeping guard. I had to stop thinking of my brother or I would lie awake all night. Quietly, I got up and found my father's rosary on the bedside table. Praying led my mind back to something that had happened earlier that week at St. Paul, my elementary school.

It had been last period of the day and hotter than hell in our classroom. We were reciting the rosary. Sister Mary Gerard sat at her desk, fighting sleep like God's good foot soldier. It was her last year teaching and we'd exhausted her. By the end of the third decade of the Glorious Mysteries, she was snoring loudly and it was not so glorious to see her lips flapping with each exhale. Some of the less holy boys and girls used this break to play tic-tac-toe, fortune teller, or hangman. Not me. I believed in the power of prayer and set all my intentions on praying Billy well.

"Hail Mary, full of grace, the Lord is with thee . . ."

"Teacher's pet," teased Kimberly Cooper and Valerie Dunne.

But I loved my glow-in-the-dark beads and figured they were probably jealous. Valerie sat behind me and Kimberly soon shared her seat, the better to taunt me.

"Let's play hangman," whispered one to the other, but with special emphasis on the word *hangman*. I still had no idea what they were after.

"That sounds like fun. But I don't know if I can concentrate with that smell. Eeeeeeeeeew, what is that?" The stink from my father's stogies clung to my uniform and surrounded me like Pig-Pen's dust cloud.

"It's coming from St. Kathy Frazier of the Holy Lunatics!"

I knew they knew about Billy and what he had tried to do far across the sea. All of my siblings had graduated from the same small grade school, leaving me alone to deal with the gossips. Their hateful glances burned the back of my head. I closed my eyes and mouthed my prayers silently, yet more fervently, "Hail Mary, full of grace, the Lord is with thee . . . "

Other kids had gathered—I could tell by their nervous giggles—but I refused to look at their gawking faces. I would not. After what seemed an hour but was probably only a few minutes, I felt warm breath very near. I finally peeked to see Valerie and Kimberly each leaning on one side of my desk. They shoved a sheet of loose-leaf up under my nose. It was their game of hangman with the drawing of a man dangling from a post, the noose tight around his penciled neck. They'd even managed to draw drops of blood pooling to a puddle with red marker. Below the figure were capital block letters, staring up at me:

BILLY FRAZIER

My tears splashed on the red marker, causing it to spread across the paper like real blood. I practically pushed Valerie down as I jumped up and ran to the girls' bathroom. I locked myself in a stall and sat on the toilet, crying until the bell rang and it was time to go home.

The morning after our first visit to Billy, Daddy and Danny went downstairs to the Holiday Inn's free continental breakfast, but my mother and I weren't hungry. I could barely move after so little sleep. I inched around the bathroom, old man style, and slowly unscrewed the toothpaste cap, imagining the pain of being my brother. Outside, my mother grunted and groaned as she heaved herself into her girdle. Selfishly, I locked the door. I hated helping her into that contraption, that armless straightjacket. Billy had been restrained since taking ill, and I dreaded that we might find him that way when we returned to the hospital for our second visit.

We'd already been to Saturday evening Mass, which counted for Sunday. By the time I shuffled from the bathroom, my mother was sitting on our double bed, fully dressed with her *I need to talk to you* face on, and I froze, toiletry bag in hand. I could hear kids from a neighboring room laughing and horsing around in the hall and was jealous of their freedom.

Mom patted the comforter and I got that same disappearing feeling as when we'd walked the winding, overly sunny hallways of the hospital. I sat beside her and she took my hand, also like the day before. Only this time it didn't anchor me. I was fading fast and entertained the idea of Mom blowing hot air all over her invisible girl.

"You sleepwalked last night," she said as if reporting the weather. Then she recounted how she'd awoken to the sounds of footsteps running fast, of locks turning, and of a door opening and closing— too close to be from the parking lot below. I had dashed from our room while sound asleep. She found me frantically wandering the hall in my baby doll pajamas. I muttered something about "finding him." My mother stopped me just as I placed my hand on the doorknob to some stranger's room and jiggled it.

A wave of disbelief crashed my head as I sat facing Mommy. I bit my cheek to keep from calling her a liar and worse. Her story was too awful to believe, too crazy to be true. But why would she lie? She squeezed my hand and I wished I could have pulled away. Sensing this, she grabbed my other hand with hers and pulled me to her, hugging me tightly. I was a ragdoll, her Shrinking Violet suffocating in her desperate embrace.

"I'm sorry," she was crying now, "you got this from me." I would drown in her tears. Her groping apology would drag me under like the weeds of Aunt Kathleen's lake.

Then she held me at arm's length and gasped as if remembering the most important detail. "Don't tell your father," she practically begged, "he's got enough on his mind with Billy."

A NIGHTCAP

Maybe it was because my parents were heartbroken to the point of distraction that they lost track of their youngest. At dusk one night during the summer after Billy got sick, I left our cul-de-sac with Colleen and crossed Route 9, the dangerous highway where my second cousin had been the victim of a hit-and-run. I was both terrified and thrilled at the prospect of hanging out with older, public school kids. The very kind of teenagers I'd feared just a few years earlier as they passed my bedroom window on their way to the liquor store. For once, I didn't care about being the good girl. My brother would be coming home from the hospital in a few days and this was my release, a mindless exorcism of my grief.

They were mostly strangers to me and I shuffled from foot to foot in Annie's empty barn-turned-garage before the booze arrived. Rock 'n' roll played from a black transistor, which the owner cradled selfishly, his baby. Annie was fifteen, in Colleen's class, and her single mom was away. I didn't know whether her father was dead or divorced, but her mother was young and pretty. My mom had been mistaken as my grandmother upon more than one occasion, which annoyed her and embarrassed me. In the coming years, Billy's illness would age both my parents even more rapidly. Annie's mother was a career woman and I romanticized their situation, as if they stepped out of an episode of *The Partridge Family*.

There were ten of us, evenly paired boys to girls, only I was too naive to figure that out until later. A few of the guys were in their late teens with low voices and broad chests that repulsed me. I was still twelve. The last of the day's light filtered dusty through the narrow cracks in the barn wall, and the air smelled like school around the corner. I dreaded the return to my mean class. I was entering eighth grade, my last year at St. Paul.

Several of the kids were smoking. I acted like it was nothing while secretly I was appalled to see my best friend French inhale. But if you'd have scratched even slightly at my shock you'd have found a whole lot of envy. A perfect halo of smoke settled around Colleen's dirty-blond hair highlighted with Sun-In. My dark brown mop was heavy compared to her fine Goldie-locks. She was two years my senior and, following her example, I'd worn my tightest tank top and denim cut offs.

Who wears short shorts?

We wear short shorts.

That was our theme jingle from the Nair commercial. We sang it often and childishly but there was nothing babyish about our butts peeking provocatively as we bounced along. I still hadn't gotten my period and the year before when I'd asked my mother what menstruation was, she flustered and said to go ask my sister. Patricia shared the chapter on reproduction in her biology book. I found it fascinating but remote—nothing to do with shaking my booty for all to see.

One of the eighteen-year-olds returned from a run to the liquor store with bottles of Boone's Farm Strawberry Hill wine. It was completely dark by now. I was supposed to be home. I had never tasted alcohol and was both afraid and fascinated by it. I knew that my dad was an alcoholic but I'd never seen him drink. From eaves-dropping on my parents' conversations, I'd learned that just as Billy was showing signs of recovering, just as he'd been given some privileges, they'd received a call from the VA. He and some other patients had gotten into trouble that included drinking and fighting.

Billy had shared with my parents about the circumstances that preceded his suicide attempt in Germany. They were unsure what to believe, what was real or what existed solely in my brother's mind. He'd said that a fight over a drug debt of a few hundred dollars had broken out in the barracks. He'd tried to defend an African American soldier who was being beat up by white American soldiers. One guy smashed a beer bottle and then dug the sharp end into Billy's head, nearly killing him. The young man who owed the money was stabbed to death. Once in the hospital, an intense paranoia gripped my brother and he feared for his life. He believed that the dealers who had killed the young man were coming to get him so he might as well do it himself. He slit his wrists.

I vowed I would never do drugs. But alcohol wasn't a drug, right?

Colleen sensed my fear when the Boone's Farm arrived and whispered to me, "It's so sweet, Kathy, you're gonna love it!"

My anxiety heightened as one kid unscrewed the wine bottle cap and took a long pull. The others hooted and transistor boy cranked up the music. "Lucy in the Sky with Diamonds" came on and we talked loudly about how cool it was that one of the girl's last name was Lennon and the tragedy of the Beatles' breakup.

"Yoko's a motherfucking bitch." The runt of a kid who said it spat to make his point. I'd never heard anyone talk that way about a woman and I felt my body seize up with fear, weighted to the spot, immobilized.

The whole gang laughed their way to the deserted sand hills between Annie's development and Route 9 and I fake-laughed along. There was a streetlamp's yellow light and blinking, flashing reds and blues from Hoffman's Playland, the rinky-dink amusement park across the two-lane highway. When the bottle came around the circle, I drank one long gulp and then coughed hard, which made the big kids laugh.

My sensitivity to the stuff was so strong that I kept blacking out even though it was my first time. It was like falling asleep while moving around and then waking up in some surprise situation. It was not unlike sleepwalking, although I made no such connection at the time.

I found myself suddenly alone behind a pine tree with the guy who'd trashed Yoko Ono. We were standing close and he was staring at me mean-eyed. His uneven but determined facial hair creeped me out. He was slump shouldered and skinny, like an old-man-kid. He took a long drag from his cigarette, as if for courage, flicked it to the dirt and ground it, hard, with his Converse. Then he grabbed me and kissed me, tight lipped until he darted his tongue into my unsuspecting mouth. He practically bit my lip before pushing me away, "There. Are you happy now? Are you satisfied?" Pulling a small bottle of golden liquor from his back pants pocket, he swigged a mouthful and thrust it at me. I obediently drank and then shamefully sulked after him toward the crowd. I was grateful he was a Shaker High kid and prayed there'd be no gossip about my failed first kiss at St. Paul.

Next thing I remember was waking up out of another blackout, dancing with Colleen in the center of the cheering circle. We were holding outstretched hands, leaning back and twirling fast to Blood, Sweat and Tears' "Spinning Wheel" blasting from the radio. I had to pee and somewhat remember crouching in the tall grass with Colleen stumbling to help me up, my shorts soaked in urine, which we found hysterical.

When I came out of the next time lapse, Colleen was lying in the sand passed out completely, only I thought she was dead. There was a boy stretched out beside her sliding his hands under her shirt. My heart beat frantically. I couldn't keep track of any of it. I screamed. Was I awake or asleep?

Then my girlfriend and I were wandering around Hoffman's, her arm about my shoulder, holding me up, as we giggled mindlessly through the crowds. I wouldn't remember the terrifying moment when I thought Colleen had died until several days later. I was also unaware that I'd crossed the treacherous highway in a blackout, just as I was oblivious to the myriad of possible dangers we'd survived at the hands of the older, drunk boys.

Danny's best friend was Michael Hoffman, whose family owned the amusement park. I'd had a crush on Michael since I was five. Anytime I was near him, my heart beat faster and my mouth went dry. I was mortified when he was the one to discover Colleen and me tripping about the rides. He was a ginger and I blushed almost as brightly as the color of his hair to think of him seeing me drunk. It was a single heartfelt moment of disgrace but then I must have blacked out again.

I came to with my sister Mary Ann putting me to bed. I felt light, even happy sitting beside her as she helped me into my nightclothes. I might have floated away but was not afraid, like during my visit to the psychiatric ward. It was a dreamy, easy feeling. I passed out fast, no worries about what torments my brother suffered or about his imminent return. No worries about falling asleep. Not a concern about leaving my bed.

I don't remember my parents confronting me in the days that followed. They were preoccupied and exhausted in anticipation of Billy's homecoming. Mom had suffered a severe *nightmare* that week and Dad was up nightly with insomnia. Maybe they thought it better to let a young person handle me. Maybe my siblings had hidden the incident from them.

Every once in a while, in the early years of my sleepwalking/sleep terrors, I recalled bits of an episode days later. Riding the bus to school, resting my tired head against the window pane, a memory of me bolting from bed, or screaming awake, or waking up with my heart beating to explode from my chest would come back to me—like a nightmare remembered days after the fact. That's how it was after my experiment with alcohol. Memories returned in fits and starts, interspersed with gaping black holes. It terrified me so that I wouldn't touch the stuff again for years.

HIT AND RUN

When I started at Notre Dame-Bishop Gibbons High School, it was a welcome relief. Fellow students were much kinder than in grade school, and I grew from painfully shy into a funny, well-liked girl. I moved easily between clicks, did well in my studies, and took pleasure from drawing and painting. I was sleep deprived both from worry over Billy and from fear of going to sleep and having episodes. However, I'd grown used to being tired and the strength of youth fed my denial.

During these years, Billy attempted suicide three more times. Deinstitutionalization was in full swing, Social Security Insurance became available, and he was honorably discharged from the army, making him a veteran eligible for benefits, including continued care in VA hospitals and daycare facilities.

His stays in psych wards increased in length. We feared that one day the doctors would throw away the key. My parents always wanted him home with us, safe and sound, and agreed to whatever treatments were prescribed. They included one-on-one therapy, group therapy, art therapy, occupational therapy, and a plethora of psychotropic drugs including heavy quantities of the daddy of them all, Thorazine. Doctors ordered sedatives, straitjackets, padded rooms, and (what I felt was a barbaric torture) electric shock treatments, now called electroconvulsive therapy (ECT). There were almost a dozen series of administrations and Billy would be returned to us docile, empty, blank.

I wanted my brother home yet secretly felt relieved when he was away. I invited friends over less and less when he was around. Guilty and confused by my feelings, I spent many sleepless nights in worry and shame.

My sisters left. Patricia married in 1972 and Mary Ann a year later. Standing at our living room picture window in the summer of 1973, I watched Mary Ann and her sweet groom, David, disappear up the hill of Glennon Road in their car and I wept. Why couldn't they take me with them?

One autumn into winter, Billy suffered a long spell of depression while locked away. It seemed to me that the grown-ups distained his despondency with a vehemence that repulsed them. They made effort to bolt it from his system. He received a series of shock treatments and was sent home in time for Christmas.

I babysat him, unofficially that is. Memory loss and confusion were side effects and I couldn't bear to leave him alone in our living room, which I'd started calling our dead room. By this time, we had two La-Z-Boy recliners. All of us alternately shared the new one by the picture window except for Billy. He preferred the worn one tucked in a corner, a shadow of the first. He shook and dosed for hours in that chair. He shook so badly I thought he might shake apart. Slowly his concentration returned. Then he smoked and read.

Piles of books towered around him on the floor, sentinels against his deadly thoughts. He made a mighty effort to tame his voices, to wrangle them and replace them with the words of Faulkner, Austin, Dostoyevsky, but could they save him? He gave me my love of literature, and I alternately read by him and sprayed Lysol—that's how much I hated the sickening cloud of cigarette smoke. Or maybe my efforts to disinfect only gave me some illusion of control.

"Grandma Tallmadge got them," my brother told me as he awoke from nodding off. It was late at night and we'd been reading by the Christmas tree. Danny and Mom and Dad had gone to bed.

I put down *Little Women*, sad to leave the safety of the March's home. I'd no idea what he meant about Mom's mom. "Grandma Tallmadge got what?"

"Shock treatments," he slurred as he lit up another Lucky, "only no anesthesia . . . back then. Surly attendant sat on her chest . . . restraining our Grandma."

I bit my lip to keep from crying.

"I'm lucky . . . I guess." Then he nodded off again. I removed the cigarette from between his fingers quietly so as not to wake him and so he wouldn't set himself—and in turn, all of us—on fire.

Dan and Billy had continued to share a room upstairs and I'd taken my sisters' old room across the hall. The spare bedroom on the first floor became where Dad pieced puzzles in the middle of the night. He loved making sense from the thousand disparate fragments.

I didn't have the strength to usher my brother up to bed and was afraid to go to my own. I put a blanket around him and settled onto the couch with another. I stared at our lights. They were supposed to give you hope during the darkest time of the year but their twinkling seemed pointless that night. I thought about my grandma, who had died when I was a baby. I thought about my brother snoring nearby. I wondered if I would be one of the unlucky ones, if I would turn out to be schizophrenic. Maybe I already was. My sleep disturbances frightened me more and more. I was especially upset from an episode I'd had on the eve of Billy's most recent return. It was the first time I woke up in the middle of sleepwalking and I hadn't dared told a soul.

In my dream, a Mac truck was speeding directly at me. My legs were braced, bent at the knees, bare feet arched against the black, burning tar of the road. Exhaust filled the air and the headlights blinded me. I felt the searing metal of the engine burn my hands, stretched out flat in one tremendous effort to stop the truck from hitting me.

In the moment of collision, I came to and the eighteen-wheeler had vanished. Hit-and-run. It was pitch-black. I was standing. I was not in bed or even in my bedroom. I couldn't catch my breath. Sweat streamed down my face and neck, and my nightshirt was soaked through. My hands pressed hard against a knotty pine wall and my legs and body were slightly bent in a pushing stance.

I stood there, frozen to the spot except for my runaway heart. All I could hear was the radiator clanking as the heat came up frantically. Some poor soul was caught in there and couldn't get out, Marley from *A Christmas Carol* dragging his chains behind him.

My eyes adjusted as the full moon broke from behind clouds and glared through the closed window. The lunacy was lost on me. Slowly—very, very slowly, I began to recognize objects. The Union and Confederate flags hanging from the wall, a worn baseball mitt slung over the bedpost, castaway scapulars and rosary beads. My heart was a punching fist and I realized then that I had been pressing with all my might against the wall of my brothers' empty room. My mind raced to locate them. Danny was away skiing with friends but where was Billy? I felt a terribly familiar feeling in the pit of my stomach. Where was my brother . . . was he dead or alive?

One frigid February night when I was fourteen, I desperately wanted to go to a friend's. I was on mid-winter break, but Billy was in a particularly manic phase—agitated, my mother called it. By this time, I'd grown even more afraid to leave him and had completely stopped bringing friends home. If only I could calm him down and get him to bed so I could go out and have some fun. This particular night, he paced the dead room with intermittent breaks to bang on the drums. They were a measure of his hysteria. He was a pretty good drummer and my parents had purchased him a set, which was kept in the basement. They hoped it would be therapeutic, but the racket was unnerving and we all fought valiantly against complaining.

That night, Dad had called down for him to stop and Billy returned to pacing in the dead room. He was full of purpose, as though he were patrolling the area. All the while, he smoked and mumbled incessantly to his invisible tormentors. He paused to perch forward in his La-Z-Boy (footrest tucked in) and enjoy his cigarette and his imaginary arguments more fully. His left leg bounced up and down nervously and ashes flew from the huge ashtray he balanced on his lap.

During this time, we'd taken in a stray, a toy poodle that more closely resembled a dirty dust mop. Billy loved the thing and it had a way of calming him. That particular night, Billy had been sitting and smoking when I approached with the dog. I felt that if I settled him with the creature, it could be a replacement sitter; maybe I could escape to my girlfriend's. He extinguished his Lucky Strike, excitedly spilling fine gray powder this way and that all over his pajamas. I was struck with a desire to bless my brother, to stick my thumb into the soft gray powder and make the sign of the cross on his forehead. It seemed a terrible waiting game, what the priest predicted each Ash Wednesday, "ashes to ashes, dust to dust."

Instead, I grabbed the ashtray from his lap with one hand and deposited it on the TV tray. The pooch had been tucked under my other arm like a football. Billy held up his hands, shaking yet open, to receive her. She flew into his arms, circled around and around his lap, and leapt up to lick his face. Even in the smoky, dim dead room, I could see it. An ease descended, and underneath his long, unkempt, Yosemite Sam mustache, Billy smiled. A real smile with teeth and everything. For that split second he was there. My before brother.

So I decided to risk leaving Billy in the care of the stray. I supervised his meds so that no accidental overdoses accidentally took place and waited until they kicked in. It was like watching an overwound toy unwind. He puttered slower and slower until he bent at the waist, head drooping. I gingerly removed his final cigarette of the day from between his fingers.

When he shuffled upstairs, the stray was cuddled inside his flannel bathrobe, a baby in a sling. He leaned heavily on the banister for support even though the dog was a tiny thing. When I tucked him in, his kindred spirit was cozy at his side, a picture of domestic bliss.

THE EXORCIST

My parents had forbidden me to watch *The Exorcist* and I'd happily complied. As both a good Catholic girl and a sleepwalker, I was terrified of possession. It was supposed to be the caviar of horror films, a whole new kind of psychological thriller. Audience members fainted. It had been banned in many parts of the world, including Ireland. It caused quite a stir among my schoolmates, but our debates were based on hearsay since none of us had been allowed to see it. One girl in my class snuck in with an older sibling. Her uncontrollable weeping at bedtime for a week afterward acted as both confession and penance. Her parents swore her to secrecy for fear of inciting other kids to see it. When begged for details, she trembled and blanched. She clamped her lips tightly and shook her head no. Some boys teased her in the halls by humming "Tubular Bells" as she passed.

Then one day I found a copy of *The Exorcist*, by William Peter Blatty in a stall of the ladies' room at the Colonie Mall. I'd held it in my hands for a long time, deliberating whether to open it. It was brand new. Somebody had obviously left it behind. To read it would be a serious sin. I'd be breaking the fifth commandment by not honoring my mother and father's orders. Or would I? They'd outlawed the movie but hadn't mentioned the book. Maybe it wouldn't be as serious as I was making it out to be, calling in the commandments. Maybe it would be considered a minor sin of omission.

I sat on the toilet and opened the book. By the time I got to the part in chapter one where the devil first raps for the mother's attention in the middle of the night, my stomach went all floppy. Chris goes to check on the noise and her newly possessed daughter is sound asleep. It's April 1 and the mom wonders if the girl, Regan, has been playing an April Fools' joke. But she is definitely sleeping. Chris decides that rats in the attic are the culprits.

Rats in the attic, bats in your belfry, a sick mind, possessed by the devil, things that go bump in the night—like me. Someone in the next stall flushed and startled me. I slammed the book shut.

Blatty was a devout Catholic. I'd heard the story was based on a real exorcism and was scaring droves of people to convert. Others said that watching it was an invitation for the devil to enter into your life. What would be my punishment if I read further? Was sleepwalking a kind of possession? And what about Billy's schizophrenia? I knew I had to read more about Regan's case.

My idea was to sneak read it, but where? I couldn't bear the thought of my parents discovering it. I worried they'd blame the book on Billy and I would not confess, sinful girl that I was, like the time I defaced the cellar door. Maybe I'd been possessed when I'd done that deed. I thought of Flip Wilson in drag as Geraldine, "The devil made me do it!" But it didn't seem so funny all alone in the confines of that stall in the bathroom of the Colonie Mall while turning *The Exorcist* over and over again in my sweaty hands.

I stuffed the book into my backpack.

That same night, and the night I left Billy in the care of the stray, my neighborhood friend Dee invited me to sleep over.

During this time, sleepwalking was always panicked, however infrequent. In an instant, I would escalate from sound asleep to fight or flight. I'd beat away or flee whoever or whatever was coming to get me. I rarely woke. Mostly I didn't remember incidents—only sometimes, like shadows of dreams, secret ghouls, cold fingers and all, to grab at my waking life. I couldn't share them over lunch in the cafeteria with my girlfriends. Slumber parties terrified me; I began sneaking drinks from liquor cabinets at friends' houses to knock myself out. Abstaining from alcohol at a sleepover made for a sleepless night or worse—like the night of *The Exorcist*.

Mr. Korzinski kept a well-stocked bar, but I decided to forego sleep completely. No booze and no sleep would enable me to avoid a sleepwalking episode and provide ample time to sneak read *The Exorcist* in their guest bathroom. I decided not to share it with my friend, afraid that I'd cave and confide about my sleepwalking. That would be disastrous because although she went to Shaker High, word might get out to my school. I couldn't have that.

That night, Dee and I watched the 1931 Boris Karloff movie, *Frankenstein*. We'd taken over the living room and spread our sleeping bags side by side, a raft adrift and floating furiously on a river of fear. Well, that's how it felt to me. Dee found the film ridiculous and was getting a kick out of my reaction. Her square, pale face, full of freckles, flickered bright and dark, bright and dark, the television light reflecting off her braces. Just as it finished, her cat jumped out of nowhere and onto my lap, humpbacked, claws digging like a Halloween cat. We screamed and then laughed but I didn't really find it at all amusing.

Above the TV, a huge tin and copper clock in the shape of a swan flying free read midnight. Mrs. K hollered from upstairs for us to be quiet. She was a working mom and needed her beauty rest.

My friend got ready for bed, but I was stuck to the spot, thinking about the soulless monster. I scratched at what was left of our Jiffy Pop stuck to the bottom of the tin and washed it down with Dr Pepper, *so misunderstood*, as the soda's jingle went. Dee returned from the bathroom, shut off the light, and whispered the three little words I dreaded most:

"Time for bed."

"Pleasant dreams," I managed.

"Same to you," she wished back as she zipped herself in for the night. I could tell by the rhythm of her breath that she fell asleep almost immediately. It seemed so easy for other people.

The plan to steal away and read my contraband was failing miserably. The movie had really scared me. Things that other kids found funny often frightened me. I hated that about myself. Now I didn't want to be up and alone all night in the Korzinski's guest bathroom. I couldn't stomach leaving my friend.

I closed my eyes and imagined what it must have been like for Dr. Frankenstein's creature. It wasn't his fault that his body parts had been dug from various graves, sewn together, and stuffed with the brain of a criminal. Two fat corks had plugged his neck to keep his head from falling off. I was terrified of losing my head, like my famous Irish relative, Robert Emmet.

One time, when Danny and I shared the downstairs bedroom, he crawled silently from his bed, hid beneath mine and waited. Just as I was dozing off, he crept up beside me and put his hands around my neck to play-strangle me. Once again, I screamed a loud, long scream, a torture movie scream. Once again, my mother boomed down the corridor and beat my brother with the wooden yardstick.

I realized then—lying next to Dee Korzinski after watching *Frankenstein*—that it was shortly after the play-strangling incident that Danny was moved upstairs to Billy's room. As Dee slept peacefully beside me, I realized that, for me, going to sleep was like being killed every night and then reanimated each morning.

I opened my eyes to remind myself of where I was. Icy light from the moon reflected off the snow and slipped through the slits where the heavy drapes didn't quite meet. The wind whistled mournfully. I reconsidered tiptoeing to their basement bar but Dee's father was a heavy drinker and hadn't yet returned from his night out at the Polish American Community Center. I was afraid he'd catch me. I preferred not to run into him at all when he was drunk, his eyes all vacant like the monster's—or like mine, my family said, when I sleepwalked.

No, I would stay put.

I'm uncertain how much time passed—an hour, maybe two. *I must be possessed*, I thought, as I quietly removed *The Exorcist* from my backpack. I turned my back to Dee, squirreled down into the sleeping bag as far as I could, and using my flashlight as a reading lamp, surrendered to my good-night story. It was hotter than hell inside that damn bag but it would have to do.

I read through the first part of the book. Chris had thrown a party and Regan walked into the middle of it while sound asleep and urinated all over the living room rug. In a lifeless voice, she told a guest who was an astronaut that he would die up there. Everybody thought she'd been sleepwalking except for Mrs. Perrin. She was psychic and counseled the mother to throw away the girl's Ouija board. She told a story about a family of eleven in Bavaria in 1921 that had held a séance. After that, they went on a burning spree. They burned up every stick of furniture in the house and then the baby. The whole family was locked away in an asylum. Mrs. Perrin warned that there are lunatic asylums all over the world filled with people who dabbled in the occult.

I had played the Ouija board with the very girl who slept soundly beside me. Why was I being singled out for punishment with my terrible sleepwalking and what about this horror in my hands? What had I done in reading it? Had I invited the devil into my sleeping bag?

What the grown-ups in the story assumed was somnambulism turned out to be possession. The very same night of the party, Regan's mattress shook uncontrollably as she begged her mother to make it stop.

It was then I returned the book to my backpack and turned off the flashlight.

Sleep seemed impossible yet inescapable. "Lights out," for me, was that inevitable moment in a horror movie when the ingénue faces a decrepit, wooden door, left slightly ajar. Innocently, she puts her hand to the doorknob, the music swells, and every single audience member silently begs, *do not open the door*. But she does. The girl opens the door anyway, as she must, and I faced the terror of my bed night after night, as I must.

I decided to lie completely still in my sleeping bag at the Korzinski's with my hands folded across my chest, pretending to be dead. I'd fool the devil himself. "I am not Regan," I whispered. I could hardly stand my sweaty feet and the elastic on my sweatpants gripping at my legs. I'd wished I'd thought to cut it away like Mom used to cut the elastic from my nightgown sleeves when I was little. As time ticked by, I worried that the Korzinski brat cat would pounce and startle me into a screaming fit, awake or asleep, claw at my exposed arms, or worse my face, so I tucked back into the bag completely and turned on my flashlight again.

The inside was flannel and patterned with a flock of brown ducks flying. I patted them with pity and envy. They were stuck, always going, never getting to rest, but at least they had each other. I hated feeling captured when I turned from side to side. Was it a little like a straitjacket? I worried that I'd left Billy at home. Tears fell upon the inside of my sleeping bag. Rain upon the family of ducks forever frozen in time.

Eventually I must have drifted off.

I woke to that panicked feeling. I'd been running from the devil himself. My heart smacked against my ribs, begging for release, and I found myself flailing. I woke to the smell of beer breath and someone's hands shaking my shoulders, hard, a gripping embrace. I was standing, or was I dreaming of standing and pounding someone's chest with my fists?

"Wake up! Wake up!" he whispered hoarsely, a demon from *The Exorcist* maybe.

His face became clear. It was Mr. Korzinski shaking me. His drunken eyelids drooped as if he would fall asleep in the middle of our struggle. We were tussling in their recently remodeled kitchen and I slipped on something wet and fell. Mr. K almost fell too but gripped the sink, laughing. His beer belly shook uncontrollably.

"Look what you did . . . to Vera's new floor . . . she's gonna kill ya . . . shhhhh," he held his finger to his lips and wiped tears from his eyes.

A yellow puddle slowly spread across the black and white linoleum. I had peed just like the girl in *The Exorcist*. Had I peed before he'd found me? Had I peed from fear of being found in that soul snatched state? But that was not the worst part. I was naked from the waist down. I must have stripped off the too-tight sweat pants while fitfully asleep inside that trap of a sleeping contraption. Mr. K handed me a dish towel to cover myself. Humiliated, I burst into tears and began my usual post-somnambulant trembling.

I ran into the guest bathroom. I couldn't stop crying but felt no real sympathy from the flamingos that flocked the shower curtain. An hour must have passed. No one came to check on me. That was a relief. Maybe Dee and her mother had slept through the incident. Maybe her father was so drunk, he wouldn't remember. I sat on the edge of the Korzinskis' pink bathtub with "Tubular Bells" ringing around my haunted head. When dawn broke, I wrapped a towel around myself, tiptoed to gather up my things, and got dressed. I cleaned their kitchen floor with my sweat pants and sprayed Lysol before sneaking out of the house. I stuffed those stupid sweats into a neighbor's garbage can but no matter how far I crammed them into the pail, I couldn't hide the evidence from myself.

Sleepwalking was a terrifyingly lonely business, sometimes more so when there were witnesses.

TOLERATE IT

After that, I rarely saw Dee, and when I did, it was only during waking hours. She never mentioned anything about my sleep-pissing or sleep-wrestling with her dad, and I blamed our waning friendship on different schools and interests. But in the winter of my junior year, Dee's sister, Elaine, who was six years her senior, gave me her December issue of *Psychology Today*.

"That's you," she said, "that's what you have." The cover tease read New Findings On: Insomnia, Sleeping Pills and Sleep Attacks and also on the cover was a photo of a man whose head had been completely shaved. Half his face was normal and that eye was closed. The other half was a pitch-black silhouette of his head and featureless except for a wide-open eyeball. The effect was startling, creepy—a modern-day Frankenstein's monster.

I felt my neck and cheeks flush. Had Mr. K squealed? Had he even remembered the incident or had he been in a sort of sleep-walking state himself, a beer-induced possession? How much of what I remembered really occurred? What had I forgotten? Elaine had been away on the night of *The Exorcist*.

"What do you mean?" I fished. I was like the alcoholic who doesn't understand that her family and friends know all too well about the drinking she made every effort to hide.

"Night terrors and sleepwalking. Be sure to read through to the end of the article." Elaine would go on to become an award-winning journalist and director of our local news. No wonder she had sniffed out the very first comprehensive article on sleep disorders published in a national magazine and had laid it in my hands. I thanked her, I guess, and, handling the periodical like I couldn't care less, stuffed it in my backpack for later that night.

It was stormy and the snow fell heavily, a pure white blanket that wrapped up our house and sealed us all in there together. I would read the *Psychology Today* piece undercover, literally under my covers, with my always-near flashlight. It was every bit as illicit as *The Exorcist*.

It wasn't drafty buried deep in my bed, but even so I felt a chill. The cover image unnerved me completely. Was I that unnatural? Obviously, yes. Howls from the wind sounded a werewolf's cry and raised the hair on my arms. I was cursed, a creature of the night. Everything terrible seems to come out after dark. The magazine shook in my hands. It took a long time to find my resolve and turn to the article.

"Sleeplessness, Sleep Attacks and Things That Go Wrong in the Night," was written by a team of five doctors from one of the first US Sleep Disorders Clinics at Stanford University's School of Medicine. It covered insomnia, sleep apnea, narcolepsy, and—tucked away at the end of the article—dysomnias, a now obsolete term that covered sleep talking, screaming in the night (night terrors), bed-wetting, sleepwalking, and teeth-grinding. "We now classify patients by the nature of their complaints: too little sleep, too much sleepiness, or behavior that upsets other people . . . Dysomniacs are obviously not paralyzed . . . abnormal behaviors come in the non-REM sleep stages characterized by slow brain waves—when the body is not paralyzed."

Dysomniac. Shameful. I'd gone to any lengths to avoid upsetting other people in my young life. Be nice, be good, be smart, my parents' pride and joy, the baby, the beauty, the apple of my father's eye, *Kathy's so quiet you wouldn't know she was here*—until night falls. My cheeks burned hot even in my self-imposed solitary confinement, but I kept on reading and rereading. I combed the article over and over in an effort to make sense of it.

Patients slept at the clinic while their brain waves, eye movements, and muscle-fiber activity were charted by sophisticated technology. Often such body processes as heartbeat, breathing, the excitability of reflexes, and the amounts of oxygen and carbon dioxide in the patient's blood were monitored. This new notion of it being, at least in part, a physical illness from which I suffered was a tremendous relief, but not for long. There was the reality of only a handful of such clinics around the world. The nearest to my upstate town was three hours away in New York City.

The sleep doctors agreed that most dysomniacs were children whose symptoms would cease by age twelve or thirteen and should be allowed to run their course. Mine had begun during early adolescence and seemed to be worsening in my teen years. In the case of an adult patient with night terrors, the team of neurologists, psychiatrists, and psychologists prescribed diazepam (a.k.a. Valium) to "suppress slow-wave sleep, stop his screams and bring tranquility to his family."

There was an awful lot of attention on how disturbing the problem was to other people. Maybe the doctors believed that the night terror patients' amnesia rendered the experience innocuous to them even while their screams suggested true terror. Here I seemed different too. I sometimes remembered the nightmare that turned into a night terror and I'd started waking more frequently in the middle of episodes, horrified. For each incident I recalled, how many had I forgotten?

In the next paragraph, they warned against the old wives' tale that the sleepwalker never harms himself—one of their young patients walked into the red embers of the family fireplace. Then the hallowed halls of medicine offered up their finest advice: "If you want to use the best practical tactics now available, you are left with controlling the victim's environment. Secure the sleepwalker in a room where he cannot hurt himself, insulate or tolerate the screams from night terrors, and change the bed wetter's sheets."

Secure the sleepwalker in a room sounded an awful lot like *lock her away in the looney bin* to me. I stared long and hard at the earnest-looking men in their little white coats in the photo at the end of the piece. "We still know so little that researchers engage in serious debate over why we need sleep, if indeed we do, and what purpose it serves."

Need sleep? I thought about my dad and his insomnia. Like most veterans of World War II, he rarely talked about all he'd endured, including D-day and the Battle of the Bulge. He'd been awarded a Purple Heart and pieces of shrapnel still floated around his body. I feared some sliver of metal would find its way to his heart. Once, he uncharacteristically confided in me that a duty of his as sergeant was to secure his men's camp each night. He'd set booby traps all around the perimeter—trip wires attached to live hand grenades—and in the mornings he'd deactivate each and every grenade-fuse. *Tricky business, that*, he'd said, and I wondered how anybody ever slept, ever, after that.

My father's turmoil over Billy's mental illness was gasoline to the fire of his insomnia. Exhausted daily and fearful of being fired, he appealed to a doctor at the Albany VA who prescribed sleeping pills. But whatever relief they initially afforded, they soon stole back, leaving my father wanting more and more while sleeping less and less. Soon they weren't working at all.

The addiction rendered him spectral, like the mother in *Long Day's Journey Into Night*. The sounds of his insomnia often floated up through the radiator vent and woke me from my own meager sleep. He'd moan and pace. He was a walking wounded and I'd imagine him wandering the fields of Germany, setting and unsetting grenade-fuses. He lost all appetite, and in photographs taken during those years, he resembles a skeleton with skin drawn over his bones. He became paranoid and accused Mom of having an affair. Then he slammed the huge sliding door to his delivery truck down on his own hand, nearly severing his thumb. After that incident, a doctor who was one of his fellow sober buddies helped him kick the pills.

To their credit, the authors of the *Psychology Today* piece had warned insomniacs against chemical dependency on hypnotic drugs, yet they seemed happy enough to prescribe Valium to the patient with night terrors. The article left me confused and angry. Why did the experts know so little about sleep? Why were so few of them working to figure it out? I'd grown to hate the psychiatrists who treated Billy. I interpreted their impotence as arrogance. Under my covers that winter night, I decided to also hate the authors of the *Psychology Today* article, but deep down in my frightened-girl heart I knew that their advice to tolerate the sleepwalking was the advice I would walk—or sleepwalk—away with. What other choice did I have? I would bear it my whole life long, like my mother before me.

Soon after I read the *Psychology Today* article, Mom and I sat in yet another psychiatrist's office discussing my brother's case. The doctor was a thin, condescending man, overworked and overwhelmed. I could tell Mommy didn't like him from her snooty face. A snubbing duel ensued. I couldn't decide which of them I hated more. The doctor asked if there was any mental illness in our family. *No*, Mom lied. She wasn't going to let him blame her genes. I was furious. Wasn't helping Billy supposed to be our mission? I disobeyed her warning glance, her *don't you ever dare share what goes on inside our house* face for the very first time and burst out that my maternal grandmother had been schizophrenic.

Later, I felt awful. Mom cried so hard, I had to drive us home. Between sobs she told me about an incident from when she was a girl. She whispered despite the fact that we were alone in the car.

She had awoken at dawn to find her mother lost, standing in the middle of their downtown Albany street during a torrential downpour. Grandma was dressed only in a flimsy nightgown and shivered uncontrollably. Gently, my little-girl-mother took her big mommy's hand and guided her away from the neighbors who peeked through curtains. Tenderly, she led her up the stairs to their flat, dried her off, and put her to bed. Had my grandmother been in the middle of a nervous breakdown or had she been sleepwalking? My mom had once confessed to me that Grandma Tallmadge also had *very, very bad nightmares*. What was the difference, I wondered, between acting crazy while awake and acting crazy while asleep? How long before I fell apart in the day instead of in the dark?

I was sent for a checkup around this time because my stomach hurt constantly. I could barely eat. The days of our family physician making house calls were long gone. I sat alone and shivering in a dressing gown in front of a strange doctor at the local medical center. My mother had wanted to join me, but I'd already begun my separation from her in whatever haphazard way I could. The doctor determined I had the beginnings of an ulcer. He was young, smart, and seemed sympathetic. He was handsome and could have been a soap opera doctor from *General Hospital*. Maybe that's why I dropped my guard and confided about my sleepwalking. His advice was, "If you're having girly troubles, I suggest you speak to your mother."

STAGE SANCTUARY

Up until my senior year of high school, I'd been the girl who could draw but secretly longed to perform. I did have an amazing memory for lyrics and my friends considered me a singer, a regular entertainer in our lunchroom lineup, but my family was worried when I auditioned for the lead in our school's musical, *Irene*. They remembered me singing off-key as a toddler. What they didn't know is that I snuck-sang at Dee's house all through my childhood. She'd bang away on their upright as I belted out "Born Free." My spirit soared.

I got the lead in *Irene*, the coming-of-age story of a plucky first-generation Irish American girl set in 1919, New York City. From the moment I stepped on stage, I felt connected to life in a way I'd never before experienced. Stage lamps with their golden-colored gels shone on my upturned face and reminded me of sunlight streaming through the stained glass windows of a church. Stage sanctuary. A full-moon spotlight illuminated my path as I strolled the proscenium. My heart beat fast and strong with every entrance. My emotion was not out of place and I wasn't too sensitive. In front of an audience, I was secure and funny, and I gave them the gift of laughter and of tears. We journeyed together to a place where time did not exist through waters of the free and unleashed heart. I'd always been chosen last for sports but finally I was an athlete, an athlete of art. The worn, raked floor was my playing field.

My favorite moment was the top of the show when the house went black, before the curtain was raised. The music soared as the bandleader, Mrs. Peterson, flailed her arms wildly. Her baton beat up and down and side, and up and down and side. The overture sailed through the instruments like in *Fantasia*. She seemed to catch the songs with her baton and fling them wildly. The packed house became electrified.

When the curtain flew skyward and we actors flooded the stage, I could almost see the music enter the audience members' ears, run through their bodies and out their feet. It became a fuse along the floor, under the stage and up through the empty space used to store metal folding chairs. It seared through the wooden floor and burned at my feet. I was walking the boards and was bitten. The bug—more of a fairy—brightened my heart like pictures of Jesus with his heart aflame.

Music flowed freely from my voice filling the gym. It drove away the ghosts of graduated basketball players and called forward apparitions of actors and storytellers, famous and unknown, ancestors and strangers who guided me as they danced with glee in the space between the audience and the auditorium's high ceiling. I wouldn't have admitted to witnessing the happy attack of the fairy spirits to my cast members or to anyone else for that matter—well maybe to Billy, but sadly he was in the hospital and would miss my performances.

The power even streamed out the top of my head, a halo divine, but it didn't stop with me because it didn't belong to me. It was bigger, older, ancient, and new all at the same time and it arced back to the orchestra and to the audience to complete the glorious circle of light.

Like sleepwalking, I'd entered an altered state of consciousness, but unlike sleepwalking, I felt fully alive and the opposite of a freak. I was in blissful communion with the hundreds of people sitting in rows of aluminum folding chairs before me. Their faces were a sea of whitecaps bobbing in the darkness and they swayed ever so slightly as I sang. For the first time in my life, I was completely sure of myself.

I even loved the grease paint as it melted down my neck. I loved the look of it, gaudy on the features of my fellow actors with our red lips, white highlight under our eyebrows, bright blue eye shadow, and our brows thickened into two dark arches, giving us each a look of being permanently startled. We were acting, acting, acting and, finally, our families were our captive audience and had to listen to us.

One night during the height of my reverie, a stagehand waved at me from offstage as he loosened the soft backdrops and they billowed like sails. I winked to him, *full speed ahead, matey*. Maybe I'd found my home on that old ship of a stage. I thought about my paternal grandmother who had crossed the sea, all alone from County Westmeath, to be a domestic servant in 1902. She wasn't much older than I was at the time, all the while knowing most girls never returned. Their villages held wakes for those who left.

I was only seven when Grandma Mary Josephine O'Connell Frazier really died. Her motionless body in the satin-lined casket, especially her arthritic hands, folded and entwined with her favorite crystal rosary, had impressed me. The work she'd done with those hands had afforded passage to America for many relatives. Safe passage for all. Well, almost all. She couldn't bring over her favorite brother because he'd inherited their family blacksmith business. Even though she was the eldest—one of the strongest people I'd ever met and could have easily shoed horses—he was the oldest boy. The great wide sea divided them forever.

When I was Irene, I left this world behind and I loved it, even while I felt guilty because I couldn't bring Billy along. I would never admit it to my fellow thespians at Notre Dame-Bishop Gibbons High School, but I silently prayed before each performance, dedicating it to him. Still, it didn't seem enough. Although it wasn't a physical ocean, the watery gulf that kept me from my brother was just as real to me as the Atlantic that had separated Grandma Frazier from her own.

As far as I know, I hadn't suffered a single night terror or sleepwalking episode throughout the rehearsal or run of *Irene*. But after it was over, I could hardly sleep at all.

SNAKE TERROR

Billy continued to be away and with graduation I was heart-broken to part ways with the best friends I'd ever had. I cried easily that summer and grew ever fearful of becoming schizophrenic. I knew it was hereditary, could come on suddenly, and well into a person's young adulthood. Surely, it was only a matter of time until my nighttime hallucinations happened during the day. I avoided bed. With all that staying up, I didn't have the opportunity to process my normal teenage angst through rest and dreaming, let alone my greater fears. Also, I'd no idea that sleep deprivation could bring on episodes.

Into July, there was an oppressive heat wave. We still didn't have air-conditioning in the upstairs bedrooms and the escalated temperatures made the prospect of bed even more unbearable than usual—if that was possible.

One hot night, after tossing and turning for hours, I decided that I'd sat in enough psychiatrists' offices to diagnose myself: I was smack in the middle of a nervous breakdown. I only wished I had my prescribed cure, a long pull off a bottle of Jack Daniels. My mom once told me that her mother had been administered a glass of brandy medicinally at bedtime to help her sleep. I was sad that mine was a dry house.

I must have eventually fallen asleep because I awoke to something weighty slithering up my calf. I threw back the sheet. It was a black water snake, like the ones I'd imagined while nearly drowning in my aunt's upstate lake. I screamed and swiped at it furiously, hurling myself to the hardwood floor. I ran from my bedroom, flung open the landing door, and missed the first step. I came to, out of the sleepwalking/terror, with my arms open wide and reaching. Danny was running up the stairs, two steps at a time, a cigarette clamped in his mouth, no chance to extinguish it. The utter look of terror on his face belied his supposed calm. His arms were outstretched, poised to catch me. We were flying trapeze artists, costars of the Frazier Family Clinically Insane Circus Act.

Dan had been on break from Northeastern University, watching late night TV, just home from carousing with high school buddies. My horror film screech had roused him to action. I'd been falling with enough force to knock over a dancing bear, and here he was, a drunk, college kid. He carried me up the stairs, deposited me on my bed, and turned on the overhead light. I frantically searched for the snake which had, of course, disappeared. My heart banged a circus-drum beat and I felt faint. I leaned over to let the blood rush to my head.

Applause blasted from the television in the dead room below, an ovation for Danny's heroism. Now both my brothers had saved me from my shadowy depths and from the snakes that resided there. I sat up and the trembling began. Danny asked me if I was all right as he drew a well-deserved drag from his Marlboro. A reward for his Marlboro man act. I shook my head no. My throat was so sore from screaming, I couldn't speak and held out my hands to show the shaking.

By this time, my parents had dashed up the stairs. They'd been enjoying a rare night of good sleep, and even in my altered state I felt my face flush hot, ashamed to have awakened them. "Dysomnias . . . behaviors that upset other people." They surrounded me, hugging me, patting my hair, back, arms, and hands as if to ground me, in an effort to bring me back to this world. Mommy's face was wet with tears and I felt sad to have added to her heartache.

Dad whispered a prayer over and over again, "Oh, my God! Oh, my God!"

"She was sleepwalking, she was sleepwalking." My brother stated the obvious twice and then the unspeakable truth: "She would have fallen down the stairs if I hadn't caught her."

My mind froze right there on the spot.

I busted out crying and grabbed my mother's hands with both of mine. I rocked back and forth on my bed, helpless. I was a weakling girl smack in the middle of a self-diagnosed nervous breakdown, my hyper-vigilant mind gripping, gripping for an answer. My father turned on every lamp in my room, on the landing, and in Danny and Billy's room across the hall as though the light might cast out our fear of impending doom. I let go of my mother's hands and held out my trembling ones, once again, to drive home the point they already knew—I was falling apart. If I could have spoken, my words would have been those of the possessed girl in Blatty's book, begging my mother to make it stop.

Suddenly I felt completely exhausted, as if the Sandman had walloped me over the head with a sack of sand. This feature of my sleep disorder reminded me of scenes from old variety shows when a hypnotist would snap his fingers in his subject's face and she'd instantly drop her head, falling under his command. I couldn't keep my eyes open one more minute, nearly careening from sitting up into my bed. No fear left, the episode had exorcised it completely. Mom tucked my top sheet in tightly in hopes of keeping me in place. As I let go, I distinguished her voice as if from a great distance. "Everything is okay now, Kathy. Everything is fine."

TRAITOR

Something broke in me after nearly falling down the stairs in the throes of a sleepwalking/night terror episode. I was not aware of the chasm in my psyche at the time—only of my uncontrollable and overwhelming desire to push everyone away. I completely denied the potentially fatal incident. Maybe denial was the only way to have kept functioning. The propensity to run for my life while sound asleep simultaneously put me at risk and left me with a shameful, guilty feeling. No matter how I secreted away my sleep disorders, they seeped into my waking life. My shadow stalked me and left me on the run, on the lamb. I was fundamentally faulty. No matter if I blamed my family and left them—no matter who I blamed or fled, I could not flee myself. It was an excruciatingly lonely place to be at the age of seventeen, which is why I buried all of those feelings like I'd imagined my broken heart buried so many years ago in the foundation of our home.

I was lucky enough to be able to turn my attention to acting. Like during my experience in my high school play, art would again buoy me. I interned during my freshman year of college with an educational theatre, The Empire State Youth Theatre. We opened The Egg, our home, and the Performing Arts Center in Albany's Empire State Plaza. We traveled New York, bringing residencies to elementary and high school students. My mother had fanned my flames of desire by cutting an audition notice from the *Knickerbocker News*. I hadn't known to memorize my monologues and ended up reading them to the artistic director, Pat Snyder. Still, she recognized my yearning and I'd found my tribe. I've always thought of the theatre as the Island of Misfit Toys in the TV Christmas special *Rudolph the Red-Nosed Reindeer*—each of us escaping our own Abominable Snow Monster to find refuge among fellow castoffs.

I performed often and took a turn with every technical job from costume construction to hanging heavy lamps. The work left me exhilarated during the day and exhausted at night. It was the kind of tired reminiscent of my pre-somnambulant days, a happy fatigue from nonstop physical play. My family reported sleepwalking incidents but they were minor, laughable compared to my flight down the stairs. And laugh we did, a kind of gallows humor, which is certainly one mask of tolerance. Mostly we made every effort to avoid the topic. During this time, I remembered next to nothing about episodes. I both hated and appreciated the amnesiac aspect of my illness. I despised feeling out of control, the uncertainty of whether I'd sleepwalked or not, but didn't miss waking up trapped in the middle of some self-constructed horror show.

I began sleeping with my door shut as a deterrent from leaving my room. Silly, since the closed door on our second-story landing hadn't stopped me on the night of my fall. I couldn't secure myself further because ours was a lockless house. Mom had banned them after one of the older kids got stuck in the bathroom as a toddler. But when I was a girl, a lock hadn't stopped me from easily exiting the dead-bolted room of the hotel while sleepwalking. I thought about asking for one to be installed on the outside of my door that my parents could operate it, but was petrified of fire. My paternal grandmother had awoken once during the middle of the night to flames licking through the ceiling above her bed. She was alone in her flat in Albany, both sons away fighting in World War II. It was the middle of winter and she narrowly escaped in her bare feet.

No outside lock was a relief in more ways than one. I also didn't want to be stuck in my bedroom with the monster I'd become in the middle of the night.

The pleasure and physical rigor of my internship somewhat tempered the insomnia. The actors were teaching me relaxation techniques. After getting into bed, I'd follow my breath and imagine the different parts of my body becoming heavier, letting go. But there was the inevitable moment when my mind would grip, seize up with fear, and my body would jerk awake.

Our troupe was scheduled to tour Italy and Israel. I was terrified to share a hotel room. In Rome, I drank to squelch my fear and woke in the middle of the night to the sympathetic face of the artistic director as she leaned over me. I was tucked into bed, her cool hand checking my perspiring forehead. I could tell she'd been summoned to assess the situation. But was she attending to me because I'd been drinking or because I'd been sleepwalking? I acted nonchalant while frantically searching for clues. There was a basin on the floor beside me, in case I vomited I surmised. That's all I recall and must have either passed out again or swooned into a post-somnambulant sleep. The next morning I cautiously asked my roommate. Apparently, I hadn't stopped at one medicinal glass of Tuscan wine and I'd made myself sick. I was relieved, preferring to be seen as a young dipsomaniac than a young dysomniac.

I did not drink again and a few mornings later, my roommate disclosed to a group of our company around the breakfast table how I'd run from sleep the night before as if the bed was on fire. She'd heard that it was dangerous to wake a sleepwalker so she talked to me gently and successfully ushered me back to bed. My face flushed red as she described the incident. Thank goodness I hadn't fought against her or acted out another scene from *The Exorcist*. Everyone was worried, but I assured them it was nothing, even bragging that I'd read about my maladies in *Psychology Today*, as if self-knowledge trumped danger.

I cajoled them into seeing it as trivial, even funny. Before I knew it, they were sharing humorous anecdotes of their families' and friends' sleepwalking. One of the techies acted out *The Honeymooners* episode when Norton sleepwalks in search of his long lost dog, Lulu. In that moment, I remembered how my family had compared me to Norton the first time I sleepwalked—only I'd had my eyes wide open. I could almost hear Billy's voice, "Like your soul had been snatched . . . like in *Night Gallery*."

My attention was brought back by laughter from the Italian waiters. They were hysterical to see the techie bumping about the restaurant, arms outstretched in the universal sign for nocturnal wandering. I felt sick to my stomach but forced myself to howl the loudest, thus adding false bravado to my toolkit of denial.

In 1978, my mother was diagnosed with cancer and underwent surgery to remove her left breast. She was fifty-eight years old. Her sister had already had a radical mastectomy. Their mom had a double mastectomy some years before she died in 1959. I found out about my grandmother's operation after my mom took ill. I wondered if Grandma Tallmadge suffered shock treatments after her surgery but couldn't bring myself to ask. The fact of some attendant sitting on her chest was terrible enough to think about, let alone the possibility of such a violation after the removal of both her breasts.

I hope I was kind toward my mother during her first fight with cancer, a good daughter. I've blocked so much of that time from my memory but can easily recall the feelings. I felt underwater once again, powerless to ease a loved one's pain. To be blossoming while she was distressed left me guilt ridden. I'm afraid that I spent most of my time at the theatre or in the company of my first serious boyfriend, Michael Hoffman—the same Michael Hoffman who had discovered me at the age of twelve, drunk and wandering his family's amusement park. He'd been Danny's classmate at St. Paul and his best friend forever, which is how long I'd had a crush on him.

Growing up, Michael was a red headed, freckled faced, run around of a kid who lit up any room he entered. He had cystic fibrosis. Back then, most children with CF didn't make it through their teens, but Mr. and Mrs. Hoffman had the resources to send Michael to Children's Hospital in Boston regularly. Buildup of mucus in his lungs led to dangerous infections. At the hospital, he'd lie on a tilted surface with his head downward on his stomach, back, or side, depending on the section of lung to be drained. A nurse thumped his rib cage to help loosen the secretions. It was painful but I only knew that by reading about it. Michael never complained. Exercise was also key in combating the disease and by the time we courted, coughing fits aside, he was a strapping young man, a golfer and skier.

We packed in all the fun we could, racing around the Berkshires in his red sports car, eating at fancy French restaurants, and pretending we had all the time in the world. Michael worked at his family's golf shop and we spent hours there talking. His German shepherd, King, guarded us and warmed our feet. I confided everything, save the sleepwalking.

It was the first time I shared openly about my brother's mental illness and my mom's cancer. Maybe because he walked with the knowledge that he'd be on this earth for a much shorter time than most of us, there was a light that surrounded him wherever he went. But he wouldn't talk about the CF and I never pushed him. He seemed lighter when we were together and I was grateful for my part in that relief.

We were both virgins and it was Christmastime when we decided to have sex. Michael's family was vacationing in some tropical place. I made an excuse to my parents that I'd be staying at a girlfriend's.

The Hoffmans had a beautiful, rambling, old house. Michael created a makeshift bed in front of the fireplace in their living room at my request. My plan was to stay awake all night after we made love to eliminate sleepwalking from the equation. I figured it would be easier to keep my vigil on a hard floor than in a soft bed. We'd been out to dinner and I hadn't touched a drop of alcohol. I also refused a nightcap at his house for fear of becoming drowsy.

Michael tended the fire, which was our only light aside from the twinkling tree. There was a storm headed our way and the wind picked up, accentuating how cozy we were about to become. He lay down on his back and motioned for me to join him, but I wanted to sit up and study him reclining there, his head resting on his folded arms. Even as a kid, I'd loved watching Michael—stolen glances when he played with Danny. I loved his copper-colored hair and his mischievous green eyes the best. Now we were about to lose our virginity together. I just hoped I wouldn't somehow fuck it up.

One comforter had a floral pattern and I played at picking roses for him to smell. He caught my hand when it was up close to his face, then grabbed me around the waist and pulled me on top of him, the full length of him. He turned my head to rest on his chest and I listened to the steady beat of his heart. Even though we were still fully clothed, it was almost too much to bear. I loved him so much and worried whether I could live up to the intimacy we were about to share. I'd seen my immersion in the theatre as running from my mother's illness and from my brother's too. My obsessive worry over separating from my family left me doubtful of my character. Sleepwalking confirmed my weak will. I should have been able to control it. I realized in that moment, lying heart to heart, just how terrified I was of having an episode in front of Michael. He was perfect in my eyes and I was a freak.

"Goddamn, I'm nervous," I whispered, and even with his lack of experience, he knew just what to do. He took my hand in his and whispered easy in my ear.

"We don't have to do a thing. We don't have to do a goddamn thing."

And he smiled.

I liked the way he said *goddamn* because he never really swore except to tease me about when I did. I knew he meant every word about not doing a thing if I didn't want to and it turned me on. I entwined my fingers at the nape of his neck and kissed him full on the lips, full and long. I was undone by that kiss. I turned my back on my fears and insecurities. Then we did it, well not all at once. It was sort of stop and start for a while—like the first time I drove a stick shift. But eventually we went all the way, however awkward and fumbling. The thing that surprised me most was how it left me with an ache in my chest, a bittersweet longing. I got it, why people smoked after sex in films, to try and damp down the unbearable vulnerability.

Wind rattled the windows and hard ice pelted the house as the storm that had been threatening all day finally hit us. We lay in each other's arms listening to it for a long time. At some point, King let out a miserable howl from the other room. He sounded like a locked away ghost, a banshee when death is near. I thought of my mother crying out in the middle of her night terrors. I thought of my own. Then the wind joined the dog's cry in stirring up the house and rattling the windows, and I felt like Dorothy caught in her house in *The Wizard of Oz*, caught and spinning helpless in the black-and-white tornado.

"Wow," I said.

Michael shushed me. "It'll quiet down soon and he will too. You're safe with me."

He dozed off then. He seemed to slip so easily into sleep and I remembered lines from a Tennyson poem.

When in the down I sink my head,
Sleep, Death's twin-brother, times my breath.

His final leaving crowded me then, even while I was afraid of leaving him first. I was terrified of both being abandoned and abandoning. I was petrified of becoming a traitor. King begged release again, whimpering softly, but Michael slept on. German shepherds are famous for their loyalty. I wished I were the dog instead of the pathetic girlfriend. I couldn't even face sleep nightly; how would I be able to help my boyfriend through his impending ordeal? I didn't seem to have inherited one drop of courageous blood from my Irish ancestors. He looked awfully young asleep beside me. I decided all men turned into boys when they slept. My father did when he napped on a Saturday afternoon. Billy did when he dozed in the dead room.

I worried that Michael would suffer. I don't know how long I lay there beside my first lover, ruminating over death, dreading loss. Maybe an hour, maybe two, but I began to feel sleepy, which frightened me. I would not ruin this night with sleepwalking. It seemed the only way to avoid sleep was to go home. I sat up and reached for my clothes.

"What's up, K?" Michael roused himself, intercepted my shirt, and wrapped his arms around me. "Are you cold? Do you want to go up to bed?"

My face burned hot in reply but I couldn't speak. I shrugged my shoulder. Fear of intimacy was winning. Fear of sleepwalking was winning. I didn't want to leave him but could see no other solution. He lowered me to the comforter. My body was powerless to resist. He had this way of stroking my wrists with his thumbs that always calmed me down, but this night I couldn't stand how thin my skin felt there. My mind raced and I saw Billy's bandaged wrists after his first suicide attempt. I thought about how fragile we all are, and the reality of losing Michael loomed again, a terrible stalking shadow. I was selfish to leave him on account of my stupid sleepwalking when all he wanted was to spend the night together. I couldn't articulate a single one of my awful thoughts but the next thing I knew, I was balling like a baby.

"Easy," he whispered.

"I'm sorry." I tried to pull away.

"No," he said, "don't do that," and he eased me close, so that my ear was turned toward the steadfast pounding in his chest once more. I closed my eyes and felt myself falling down the stairs. I quickly opened them with a gasp.

"What is it, K?" he nearly begged.

Somehow I found the courage to confide that I was afraid to go to sleep. He asked me if I had nightmares but all I could do was shrug my shoulder again. "Do you?" I managed to peep.

"Sometimes," he replied just as quietly and my heart broke into a million pieces on the spot. I encouraged him to talk about it but he only shook his head no, he wouldn't.

"I'm sorry. I wish I could make it right," I said and squeezed him mightily, which always made him smile.

"Rest." He comforted me when it should have been the other way around. "Just rest, K."

Eventually I settled into his embrace. The fire was so warm on my face. The flames were mesmerizing. I must have let down my guard and dozed for a moment, only to wake with drool slipping out the side of my mouth and about to pool on his chest.

"I need you to bring me home," I whispered, nearly pleading.

"I'd like to bring you home, I'd like to bring you home every night," he answered.

A shiver went through me. Ice pelted the Hoffman house with a vengeance. No sound from the dog. He must have cried himself to sleep. Michael and I were nose to nose then. I could hardly stand the way he stared right into me. "I'm sorry to be such a baby. I'm sorry to be such a scaredy-cat," and I looked away, hoping he assumed I was afraid of the weather. He took my face in his hands, like you do to a little kid when you want to make sure she understands you fully, and he turned my face back to his own.

I let him look at me with his eyes, the color of green glass worn soft from the sea.

"Home," he said and he kissed me full on the lips. "I'd bring home my K." The wind pressed the bare trees against the window panes and Michael's arms were a boat cradling me through the storm. I could resist no longer and closed my weary eyes. I hadn't prayed in forever but found myself silently imploring— *Angel of God, my guardian dear, to whom His love entrusts me here, ever this night be at my side to light and guard, to rule and guide.*

I woke from the sound of my own screams as I thrashed about in the dark against whatever it was that was coming to get me. Had an intruder broken in? Was I was being murdered in my sleep? Michael had jumped up beside me, too, completely panicked. He wrapped his arms about me, like you'd do to a child in the throes of a tantrum. But my adrenalin was pumping as if the imagined attack was real. I was strong in my sleep and fought him.

"It's me, it's me, it's Michael."

I came more fully to, struggling there, against his embrace. When I realized what was happening, I cried from shame. He shushed me and held me and asked if I was okay. I couldn't reply because my throat had seized up from my death cries. He quickly assured me, "It was a nightmare. You had a nightmare."

My eyes adjusted quickly, even with the fire nearly gone, and I broke down completely from the relief of coming to, out of the night terror. I shivered and stuck my hands out to show him my shakes. Sweat poured forth. He wiped his hand across my forehead and I wished he could as easily have removed my disgrace. He rocked me and cooed and asked me what had happened.

I shook my head no. How could I talk about it? I had no words. All I could think was, *Thank God it hadn't been worse.* Thank God I'd woken up, especially since I hadn't been doing so lately. No, better to let him believe I'd had a bad nightmare than to confide the insanity of my truth.

The ice storm seemed as though it would never pass. "I got you," Michael whispered and he held me as close as one person could. I pretended to let him comfort me but had disappeared completely, lost in my own storm of worry and despair. Had Danny told him about my fall down the stairs? Did he think I was mentally ill? I felt mentally ill. Possessed. I repulsed myself and suddenly could not stand him near me. I couldn't stand us, skin to skin. I all but pushed him away and when I asked him again to take me home, he sadly complied.

DISAPPEARING ACT

I stayed in my bedroom for several days after abandoning Michael—refused his calls, didn't shower, and barely ate. Remorse and self-contempt kept me awake nights. I was terrified, too, of having another dangerous sleepwalking episode like the time I fell down the stairs. I would finally fall asleep with the light of day.

During this time, I'd been working as a magician's assistant. Tim Snapp was tall, slender, and sleight of hand with long, fine fingers and a pointed beard that gave him the look of a handsome, if somewhat demented, devil. Being the beautiful girl that helped him didn't pay well but felt closer to acting than waiting tables or being a cashier. He was ten years older than me and had been a company member of the Empire State Youth Theatre when I'd interned.

We had a holiday performance scheduled at a local Kiwanis Club a few days after all that had happened with my boyfriend. I'd completely forgotten about it until Tim arrived at my house to give me a lift in his dilapidated Volkswagen bus leftover from his hippie days. I woke with a start when the doorbell rang and had a sinking feeling in my stomach when I saw Tim's face at our front door. I'd been the one to answer, wrapped in Billy's old bathrobe that I'd been wearing for comfort's sake.

I couldn't believe I let Tim into the dead room but had been too nonplussed to suggest he wait in the bus. Danny was passed out on our newer La-Z-Boy from his previous night of carousing. Even the doorbell hadn't roused him. My parents were in their room reading the *Knickerbocker News* on their bed. They'd both popped their heads out and given a wave when my boss had first arrived, then quickly retreated. I was embarrassed by their social anxiety and oblivious to my own.

I hurried upstairs and dressed in my black leotard (too short for my body) and black fishnet tights (too long for my legs). They'd been stuffed in my dirty laundry bin since the last time we'd performed and stunk of body odor. The most uncomfortable and ridiculous piece to my costume, a purple sequence miniskirt, was held together by pins. My insides matched my outfit perfectly—dirty, ugly, and desperately in need of repair.

I checked on Billy, who had fallen asleep in his room reading *War and Peace*.

"Who's here, Kathy?" His breathing was labored by the tome across his chest.

"Tim Snapp. We've got a show."

"Are you gonna finally tell me how you work that disappearing trick or not?"

I mimed turning an invisible key to lock my lips. I folded the page corner to mark his place and removed the book from his chest. He hadn't been hospitalized in some months, and I felt safe enough to shut the light and the door and leave him alone to rest with Tolstoy standing guard on the floor beside him.

I shakily descended the stairs while stuffing instruments of illusion into my backpack: makeup, hairpins, falsies. Tim sat on the worn, green couch looking at me disdainfully and nervously tapping an open palm with his magic wand.

It was a gloomy, gray day. Our Christmas tree lights were the only ones on in the dead room except for flickering from the television.

Its volume was loud, but I was too tired to think of turning it down. Danny must have been watching it before he passed out. Unlike me, he never bothered to hide his drinking. In fact, he flaunted it, flailed it about—simultaneously a dare and a warning. It was how he dealt with Billy's illness, the impossible expectations of being Daddy's golden boy, and those early years as scapegoat to my mother's rage. I was ashamed of him as he snored loudly. I was ashamed of myself.

A rerun of *The Addams Family* was about to start. How perfect, I thought, as the show's theme song blared:

They're creepy and they're kooky, mysterious and spooky,
They're altogether ooky, the Addams Family.

Tim asked if he could use our phone to let the Kiwanis Club president know we would be late. I turned down the television and sat beside him on the sofa, hoping he wouldn't notice my trembling. He practically yelled into the heavy, black phone, a barker to my family freak show and happy for communication with the outside world. As he hung up, Danny grumbled in his sleep and I felt my face burn hot. Tim stared at his feet and asked if I was ready. I felt paralyzed with exhaustion and fear.

"Just need to use the bathroom," I lied.

"I'll warm up the bus. Hurry up, okay?"

He couldn't seem to wait to get out of there. As he closed the storm door, I wished I could have left my family behind as easily but was frozen to the spot. I bit my lip and swallowed the heartbreak of the last few days. I had fucked up with Michael by letting myself fall asleep after making love, by having a night terror in front of him. Or was I just a selfish girl, afraid of the trials he faced? Both, I decided. Even if he could accept me, I could not accept myself.

Danny nearly snored himself awake. His face was bloated from all the boozing and I felt a sudden and all-consuming fear of him. He'd picked up the baton of rage passed by my parents. I would never let my brother know how I broke his best friend's heart. He muttered plaintively as if he were dreaming of running away, and I was reminded of how he'd cry in his sleep when we'd shared a room. The wavering lights of the television took my attention, and my fear transformed into an aching sadness remembering how we'd shared a big chair in this very room the first time we watched *The Wizard of Oz*. We'd grasped hands tightly each time the Wicked Witch appeared. As the little kids of the family, we'd had an unspoken agreement to protect each other, but when it came to it, it was every man for himself.

The volume on the TV was still turned down. Uncle Fester laughed silently at being electrocuted and I laughed aloud, a gallows humor or perhaps a premonition. Danny began struggling awake. "What'sh sho funny?" he slurred defensively, as if I'd been laughing *at* him. His face was a ghastly shade of green and the sour smell of last night's alcohol wafted from his breath. He lit a cigarette, grunted, and gestured toward the TV. "Why's the volume down? Turn up the volume." He had a vacant look in his eyes as if he were still sleeping, as if he were sleep talking. I was suddenly repulsed by my brother and by myself. We were Thing and Cousin It.

Tim honked the horn. This angered Danny and he raised his voice, "Turn up the goddamn TV."

I felt the blood rise through my face and before I could stop myself I'd snapped back, "I'm late. Turn it up yourself." My sassy response startled me. My heart skipped a spastic beat.

"Turn up the TV, you fucking bitch." Cigarette dangling from his mouth, he jerked the lever on the recliner, the leg rest lurched away and he leaned forward, ready to spring from his seat. Danny sometimes called Mom a bitch when he'd been drinking and had been threatening violence ever since he grew too big for her to use as a whipping post. Once, his girlfriend had a black eye, which she'd said happened because of a fall. He was an abused Irish boy turned abuser and so the beat goes on.

There was a very strange feeling in my hands and arms when he called me a bitch. When we were kids, Danny and I would take turns standing in the entranceway from our hall to the dead room, pressing the fronts of both arms against the doorjamb for a minute or more. I'd pretend to be a bird caught in someone's hands trying to lift my wings free. Stepping away from the doorway, my arms would fly up, like marionette arms pulled by imaginary strings feeling heavy and light at the same time.

"I said turn up the television, bitch." He jutted his jaw forward and blew smoke directly at me. We hadn't physically fought for years, and my body moved of its own accord in answer to his dare. I stood and stepped toward him even as I seemed to be watching the scene from the corner of the room where the angel perched atop our Christmas tree. I felt the slow motion movement of my right hand swinging high behind my head, collecting force, and the great release of a hard slap across my brother's face. His cigarette flew from his mouth. I felt a great satisfaction and wished that I could have slapped away his disrespect, his drunkenness, the truth of his life, the truth of mine.

He was shocked but rose to the occasion, suddenly lumbering over me. This is how we showed our love, this dance of rage. His fist came up fast and punched me hard in the left eye as if he, too, had been waiting a long, long time for the match. Was it me screaming, "No . . . no!" or was it Mommy as she bounded from her room, Daddy right behind her?

The brawl had brought Tim to the front steps and I ran from the house, sobbing, without my coat.

"Oh, my God. Oh, my God. Oh, my God," Mom screeched from behind the slammed door.

My father followed me out of the house begging, "What happened, what happened?"

Tim understood that I had to get away, and grabbing my hand, he pulled me to the bus, which was still running. He somehow got me into the passenger seat and I'd locked the door before my father began banging on the window with an open hand, pleading for me to roll it down, but we were already in reverse and backing out of the driveway.

I leaned my head against the window and wept for I don't know how long. Good thing it was a bit of a drive to the Kiwanis Club. All I could do was worry if Billy was all right.

Eventually Tim asked gently, "Are you gonna be all right? Will you be able to do the show?"

I couldn't speak and held up my left hand in a go-away gesture. I pulled under-eye concealer from my bag along with every trick from my childhood to cease my tears and turn my wounds invisible. The thought I had when I looked in a mirror was what a stupid, stupid bitch I really was. The darkening eye was well-deserved. I decided that Danny must have known, or at least known on some level, that I'd betrayed Michael. I was most certainly a bitch. I decided there and then in Tim Snapp's dirty Volkswagen bus that smelled of old shoes and weed that I would never again love anyone, ever.

Tim turned on the radio and I was reminded by "Hotel California" that I could check out anytime I want, but I could never leave.

I did assist Tim Snapp that afternoon at the Kiwanis holiday show, shaking all the way. I'm sure I couldn't meet anyone's eye as my own swelled purple. I felt stuck in a slow-motion nightmare, weighted by the shock of the fight and by my physical and psychic pain.

The finale was a superb Houdini disappearing act—the one Billy had referred to earlier when I'd mimed at sealed lips. In life, asleep or awake, all I wanted to do was vanish into thin air, which is why I loved this trick:

Tim handcuffed me, put a sack over my head, and stuffed me into a wooden crate secured with a metal chain, locked, and checked by the picture-perfect wife of a Kiwanis member. He then climbed on top of the box while holding a curtain up around himself, the box and me locked inside. By a measured count of three, he had dropped the curtain, disappeared into the crate, and I was standing atop it, supposedly coy and clever. The audience burst into applause.

At this point, I had jumped to the floor and was supposed to present the key from my pocket with flair and unlock Tim from the crate. I just couldn't pull off the flair part this particular day. My eye, which hadn't hurt at all during the performance due to adrenaline rush, throbbed and teared. As in the bus, I bit my lip but the tears flowed. Then I held my breath in an effort to control my emotions, but none of my old tricks worked. My hands shook uncontrollably, and when I tried to locate the key to unlock the crate, it was not in the pocket of my purple, sequined skirt and was nowhere to be found.

Soon enough, the audience realized something was wrong and a hush descended. I could sense their pity. My search became frantic. I couldn't find the key. I couldn't find the key. Just like in life, I couldn't find the key. I burst out in tears and Tim burst out of the box through the secret door in the lid with a fake smile for the lodge members alternated with a real scowl for me. The young wife who had come onstage to check the chain comforted me as her husband frantically pulled the ropes off stage to close the curtains. It was like the scene in *The Wizard of Oz* when the wizard is found out to be a sham.

Despite my mistake, which would come to ruin his reputation as a magician, Tim was kind enough to drive me to Mary Ann and David's house. They had two small children but let me stay with them for the remainder of my Christmas break. I slept on a sofa bed in their basement and seriously feared the possibility of screaming awake my niece and nephew. I tried not to sleep and when I did, I often woke in the middle of a night terror, dashing for the light switch on the wall. I'd be drenched in sweat, always lost as to who or where I was. I woke to night sweats and to my heart threatening an attack, or so it seemed to me. But one symptom had changed since my fight with Danny and remained changed for a while: my scream became a silent scream. I had completely swallowed my voice.

PART II: BREAKING AWAY, FALLING APART

Gentlewoman: Lo you, here she comes!
This is her very guise, and, upon my life, fast asleep. . .
Doctor: You see, her eyes are open.
Gentlewoman: Ay, but their sense is shut.

Macbeth, by William Shakespeare

TSUNAMI TERRORS

After Christmas, I moved into a suite in a tall tower at the State University of New York at Albany for my second semester as a theatre major. Thankfully, the windows were slender and only cranked open slightly. Episodes continued. They were almost always panicked, with the recurring theme of someone or something coming to get me. I covered my fear by playing the clown. My sleepwalking was considered hilarious. Thus began a more consistent flaunting of my malady along the lines of the hurrahs when I'd sleepwalked in Italy.

I was a model student, excelled in my theatre, literature, and art history classes. I acted in lots of plays and received favorable reviews. I kept a rigorous schedule, and the strength of youth continued to help me deny my fatigue and fed my denial. Maybe I associated the dangerous aspect of my somnambulism with home, with childhood, and all I'd left behind. *If your eye be your problem, pluck it out.* College was a fresh start. Surely I would never face a flight of stairs again while sound asleep.

One semester I took the top bunk of a triple room. My roommates, both theatre majors, joked that they could tell when I was sleeptalking because my voice would boom and I'd lean over the side of the bed, gesticulating wildly. Awake, I'd speak softly and my covers were tucked in tightly, restrictively—I lay still as death. I navigated the ladder from my bunk easily while sound asleep. I'd begun to deny the danger of my own experience and dare my sleeping self.

Despite my mascot status, I could not shake the shame of splitting with Michael. I felt remorseful, too, for leaving home with my mom so soon into her recovery from cancer. And then there were my continued feelings of powerlessness over Billy's schizophrenia. He hadn't been hospitalized since August 1978, almost six months before I moved on campus. Still I worried about him having another breakdown. I felt selfish for enjoying college. My defects loomed larger in the dark.

I drank to help me fall asleep even while that method consistently failed. We were a party school and it was easy to blame the nocturnal wandering on one too many beers. The amnesiac aspect of my malady rendered me clueless as to whether I'd been sleepwalking or drunk. Come morning, I found myself at the mercy of other partiers to piece together the events of the previous evening. I was reminded of my father trying to make sense out of life from his jigsaw puzzles. Eventually I stopped my queries, knowing sense could not be wrangled from the night. With that defeat, my carousing took on a masochism that my schoolmates lacked. I itched for something I couldn't put my finger on. Recklessness turned risky when I became promiscuous, earning the ridiculous nickname Floozy Frazier. Maybe I thought to escape my stalking fear by becoming a moving target. I was like a leaf on the wind when it came to my most intimate relationships.

In a state that can only be described as sleepwalking while wide awake, I accepted a proposal of marriage in my junior year. It was my best effort to wrangle myself and prove normalcy.

Don was a fellow student at Albany State and a drinking buddy. We'd only known each other six months when he popped the question. He was the oldest of three boys with a take charge personality and a big heart—the perfect nocturnal bodyguard. I don't know how often I had episodes but remembered very few. Maybe I mistook my lack of recall for health. Maybe he mistook his wife for a hat. Don was a heavy sleeper on top of being a heavy drinker. I'd told him about the *Psychology Today* article and taught him the keystone to dealing with the architecture of my sleep problems—tolerance. It was all very, *I'm Okay-You're Okay*. Denial disguised as full disclosure. Burying my true feelings beneath my swagger became habitual. Most of the time I didn't even know how I felt. My fiancé became my teddy bear. I disliked the dependency even while I clung to him nightly.

During the final fitting for my wedding gown, I stood on the little wooden box while facing a full-length mirror. There was something submissive in the Japanese style design that had been my idea. Maybe I thought of myself as an offering to the gods of wedlock in exchange for relief from my nightly burden. I was about to become the ultimate good girl. The dress was made of silk brocade with long sleeves and a mandarin collar, but the seamstress had added a horrible tiny bow at the neck. She was French and the notion was a concession in lieu of the lace and pearls she usually lavished upon her brides. I imagined a noose around my neck and kicking the stand away. I burst out crying. My mother held me. The bow went. I only wish my emotional state could have been so easily remedied.

I hadn't suffered an earache since St. Dymphna's Day 1972, when we'd found out about Billy's first suicide attempt. But on my wedding day, July 5, 1980, I could barely stand from the pain in my severely infected right ear. It's like my body was trying to tell me the marriage was really bad news but I wouldn't listen. I acted my way through the reception on antibiotics, wine, and an adrenalin rush similar to what I commonly felt on stage or in the throes of a night terror. Afterward, the plan was to drop off the gifts at our place in downtown Albany, get changed, and drive to a B&B in Vermont for our honeymoon.

I wept on the hardwood floor of our newlywed apartment, a crumpled bride with a terrible realization pounding 'round my head, more of a feeling than a thought—those tears last week were not about the gown. It had been a church wedding in concession to my parents even though I was not a practicing Catholic. Still, thirteen years of parochial school slapped any idea of divorce from my mind as quickly as a rap from a nun's ruler. The earache felt like God's punishment and a terrible omen. I was repulsed and ashamed by my collapse.

Dreaded night was quickly approaching and so was my transformation from Dr. Jekyll to Mr. Hyde. Don was drunk and ignored my wide-awake spell by stacking boxes of gifts in the other room, but his annoyance hung wordlessly between us. A cork popped in the kitchen. A moment later, he appeared with two tumblers full of champagne. We hadn't time yet to unpack our new champagne flutes, and I thought, *This is why I married him, he knows when to pour me a drink.*

My hair had been styled into a controlled bun and I loosened it. Dozens of hairpins sprang free along with rice that had been stuck there, thrown by well-wishers. I scratched my scalp frantically like a mad dog bride. I could have torn myself to pieces from the congratulatory rice on top of the earache. I covered my ear with my hand as another piercing pain shot through my head. Still on my knees, I threw my head back and howled, begging the rising moon for relief. Sometimes Mr. Hyde was depicted as a werewolf.

My groom, more tender now, passed me the champagne and I drank it like water. He squatted beside me and patted my head. I wiped my mouth with my paw. He stood then and shook his head in disgust. Don was over six feet tall and I wrapped my arms around his leg, clinging to his tux pants and whimpering. He remained still as a statue, arms crossed, staring at me with his beautiful green eyes and admonished disdainfully, "What's it going to be? What do you want, Kathy? Do you want to go on our honeymoon or do you want to go to the hospital?" He meant the ER, but images of psychiatric wards appeared before me. I thought to answer, *Take me to the mental wing of the hospital where I belong for marrying while sound asleep,* but instead I hung my head and sobbed, "Honeymoon." I couldn't dare joke aloud about the psych ward. My fear of being committed was too real.

The next year and a half passed as if in a dream. We played at husband and wife, yet my malady wore on our relationship. Daily, I denied it but nightly my shame mounted. For him it was, well, exhausting—like an extended game of Russian roulette. Would he pass a peaceful night beside me or wake to a zombie from *Night of the Living Dead*?

After graduating from college, I was accepted to Circle-in-the-Square Theatre School. Don took a job in Manhattan at the West Side YMCA managing their adult education program and we moved to Fairview, New Jersey, across the Hudson from the city.

I felt a creative kinship with my fellow actors and teachers that had been missing in my relationship. I began to discover myself as an artist. Throughout college I'd set my sights on professional training, but I was unprepared for the complete refuge I felt upon my return to the Island of Misfit Toys. The program was eclectic with teachers from Yale, Broadway, and The Actors Studio.

Two brilliant members from the Studio, Terry Hayden and Jackie Brookes, taught us to sift for actors' gold through Affective Memory and Private Moment exercises. Our bodies were our instruments, our psyches—our palates. Art took us by the hands and introduced us to the deepest, richest wellsprings of our humanity. The work both fascinated and daunted me. Unwittingly, I investigated events that had fueled the sleep disorders. Intuitively, I sidestepped the episodes themselves. I was unwilling to go there for fear of falling into the center of the earth, never to return. It was scary enough as it was.

The trip was all-consuming, but Don was not along for the ride. Despite him being a good audience member and my number-one fan, I began to see us as college sweethearts, something from the past. I had that guilty feeling again, like I was about to leave another someone behind. I was twenty-two and the only married student at the theatre. My mistake was becoming more and more apparent.

The first weekend of December 1981, we were visiting Don's parents in Rockland County when Billy telephoned from home. It had been three years since he'd been hospitalized and I worried that he'd gone out of his way to reach me, calling my in-laws when the answering machine had picked up at our apartment. I could tell something was wrong from the sound of his voice.

"I'm sorry, Kathy, I'm sorry, Babe." I imagined slit wrists and emptied pill bottles.

"Are you okay, Billy, are you all right?"

"I'm sorry, Kathy. I'm so sorry . . . we forgot to call you, Babe . . . and when I realized, I just felt terrible, Kathy . . . I had to find you right away. Michael Hoffman died. He died on October 2, Kathy . . . Feast of the Guardian Angels."

I felt miles away from everyone, like when I was a kid with a dangerously high fever. I could see faces before me; I could hear their voices, but everything was distorted and dreamlike. It was like waking up in the middle of an episode.

I came out of the shock sitting on a hassock in my in-laws' living room with a drink in my hand. Don sat beside me, holding my other hand. The pain in my heart was like a bird caught there and beating its wings furiously to break free. No matter what condolences were said to me, no matter what kindnesses shown, all I seemed to hear was Michael's voice whispering above the banshee cry of his dog and the winter wind, "I'd like to bring you home, I'd like to bring you home every night."

The next week, I holed up in our apartment, too vulnerable to go out, let alone into Manhattan for classes. But I did not cry. I wished I could, but all I felt was the weight of that dead bird where my heart should have been. I was grateful when Don left for work each morning. It was a relief to stop pretending that I would be all right—that we would be all right when I knew we wouldn't.

Don was a marathon runner and had tried to interest me but I'd hated running. Once, during our engagement, we'd been jogging the perimeter of the Albany State campus. I exhausted quickly and slowed to a walk. Neither of us realized the severity of my fatigue. I was tired all the time from fear of going to sleep whether I had an episode or not. "You never finish anything," he scolded. "How are you going to stay married when you can't run more than a mile?"

He'd found my Achilles heel. I hadn't been able to stay the course with my first real sweetheart, why would I be able to keep my commitment to our marriage? These were the thoughts that swam in my head as Don lay beside me the week after the news of Michael's death. He slept soundly, but I was repulsed by the idea of letting go to that intimacy. I was repulsed by myself. Once he'd drifted off, I'd rise—do anything to keep myself awake. I drank coffee by the pot full.

In the middle of one night, I snuck out of the flat to walk the deserted streets. It was an Italian neighborhood, residential, but that didn't mean it was safe. I wore my Walkman—oblivious to my surroundings. I played "Walking After Midnight," repeatedly. I was lonesome and searching. It was cold and I stopped to stare into Pedoto's Bakery, wishing for an espresso to both warm me and keep me up. Right there at my feet was a pack of Lucky Strikes—Billy's brand. I'd heard that nicotine was a stimulant. I picked them up. Whoever dropped them had been kind enough to include matches tucked inside the box.

I rolled the cigarette between my nervous fingers. Why had I hated Billy's smoking so much as a kid? I couldn't think of one good reason, lost as I was in the middle of my heartache. I held it to my nose and fell instantly in love with the smell of tobacco. Just like old TV ads insinuated, it smelled like the promise of something truly rewarding. That cigarette smelled like relief.

"Goddamn," I said to the dark. I almost heard Michael's voice teasingly reply, "Goddamn." I poised to strike the match and glimpsed my image in the bakery window. I'd always had such a baby face, but the cigarette dangling from the corner of my mouth destroyed that sweetness. I could hardly contain my glee. I hoped to become a bad girl, for real.

I lit up.

I was expecting the romance of the old black-and-white pictures my mom and I used to watch on television . . . *Dinner at Eight*, all the *Thin Man* series, and *Casablanca*, too. I was expecting to see the stupid girl in Pedoto's window transform into a glamorous movie star, sure of herself—like Barbara Stanwyck—with a smart mouth and all the answers. Instead I coughed up a chest-full of crap on the empty sidewalk. My lungs were on fire and the crazy thing is—I liked it. Finally something reached me. If I was too stoic to cry then maybe the cigarette would act as a tonic to clear my grief. I took another puff and another and another until I calmed down. I decided I could get the hang of being a bad girl, I could.

During the days, I dozed. Just like when I was a kid, I never sleep-walked or had a terror while napping. But those meager rests could not sustain me. I was starting to see the connection between sleep deprivation and more frequent sleepwalking. It was only a matter of time. Maybe some part of me longed for the release of emotion that always came with an episode.

One night, toward the end of that week, after lying awake for hours while Don snored softly beside me, I rose. Too exhausted to go walking after midnight, I tiptoed into the kitchen and turned on the radio—the volume low. Tuesday had been the first anniversary of John Lennon's death and the DJs continued to air tributes. "Woman" played. Plaintively, he begged Yoko to hold him close to her heart. He sang that distance could not keep them apart. I almost felt Michael beside me. I'd cried when my favorite Beatle had been murdered the year before and finally fell apart with the impossibility of my loss on top of the shame of having abandoned Michael.

Once the tears started, I feared they would not stop. This had always been the way, and it frightened me. If Don discovered me in this state, would he think I was having a nervous breakdown? Was I having a nervous breakdown?

One morning when I was a teenager, a robin flew into our picture window. It was during the height of Billy's illness and my father and I were both exhausted from insomnia. He hoped the bird had only been stunned and picked it up. It fluttered weakly in his huge hands. This set me crying. It was an indulgence that I had forbidden myself for some time and that my father could not stand. I held my breath and even pinched myself to try and stop, but I couldn't.

He brought the bird to the backyard, stood on the top of the hill, and released her to the fields behind our property. "If it wants to live, it has to fly." There were wild cats back there behind our house. When she plummeted and disappeared into the tall reeds, I sobbed out of control. My father grabbed me by both shoulders and looked me in the eye, pathetically. "You can't go crying over every little thing."

I was still that pitiful girl, secretly weeping at the kitchen table. My head rested on my arms, like during naptime in kindergarten. I began to calm down and sleep threatened. I decided to sneak-smoke in an effort to rouse myself. I cracked a window slightly and pulled up a chair with my head against the cold pane. Only planets were visible so near to the city; still I wished on the first I noticed. As a child, I had begged true love from each night's first star. But there was nothing true in how I'd treated Michael.

I must have closed my eyes because I woke to a hot sting to my leg. I thought it was a bee—a night terror bee—and swatted madly at it. As I came to, I realized that the cigarette had fallen from my grasp and landed on my bare thigh. Maybe it wasn't the safest stimulant. My hands trembled. Relieved that I hadn't screamed and woken Don, I disposed of the extinguished butt in a glass of water. It floated around, turning it sooty and gray—just the way I felt. I flushed the evidence down the toilet. Defeated, I crawled into bed.

I forgot to mention that we slept on a water bed. We thought it'd be cool, but being physically startled from sleep could initiate an episode. Sometimes when my husband tossed or turned—all 185 pounds of him—I crashed awake like a skiff against a rocky shore.

On that night when I finally gave in to sleep, I dreamt of being cast about the ocean all alone in an ancient, wooden lifeboat during the worst of a storm. Wind howled, rains railed, and thunder boomed as lightning lit the blackened sky. Bitter water filled the boat in gushes. I crouched on the floor and clung to the splintering seat until a great wave swept me away. I went under and then emerged. I struggled for air. Then something wrapped around my limbs. They were eels and the water was suddenly full of them. I beat my hands against the sea in an effort to free myself but the more I resisted, the tighter they coiled, especially around my wrists.

I woke up screaming and flailing, restrained by my husband, who was at first unrecognizable to me. He yelled, "Stop it. Stop it. Wake up. Wake up," and had responded instinctively to my attack by gripping my wrists. His fingers exacerbated my fear of the eels. I guess you could say that his fingers *were* the eels. The terror on his face was a reflection of my own.

Don held me, but the gulf between us had widened beyond all measure. Or maybe our relationship had reached a vanishing point. I could not get the image of his desperate face out of my mind. It haunted me. I worried that I was broken beyond repair. I felt both trapped by and less than my husband. My fear of being involuntarily committed to a psychiatric hospital grew considerably.

I began calculating a preemptive strike, pushing Don away by nearly turning rehearsals for a love scene into an actual dalliance. Then came the night when we got drunk with a college friend who stayed over. We'd both orchestrated the situation, yet I took the fall. I fell from grace—all too anxious to assume the role of scapegoat. Within months, I left for good.

WITCHCRAFT

I found myself alone in the city that never sleeps. Don had left the few belongings that I'd brought into the relationship on the landing outside our apartment and locked the door. He was intentionally out when a couple of actors from school helped me move my things. I walked away from the marriage unencumbered by possessions but my guilt had stockpiled.

According to my Catholic upbringing, I was an adulteress, and would be, even after Don and I legally separated and later divorced. I had violated the Ten Commandments. It was also a mortal sin, meeting all three criteria of being a serious matter, premeditated, and executed under my own free will. Confession and a firm resolve to quit the sin could have restored me to God's saving grace, but I had no such intention on either count. I considered those dictates archaic and misogynistic. Although I may not have believed in God, I sure as hell believed in hell. My own thoughts stoned me nightly.

It was well into the second semester of my first year at Circle-in-the-Square when we separated. I threw myself into my art. After classes and rehearsals, my colleagues and I gathered regularly at the dives in Hell's Kitchen to discuss our work. I was homeless and couch surfed, dependent on friends' kindness to buoy me through my breakup.

One night, a group of us met at the Film Center Café. Discussion led to Arthur Miller's *The Crucible*. We understood the play was an analogy for McCarthyism. We debated power, playing on people's fears, and mob mentality. Somebody said the Salem witch hunt had been a pretense to gain land. We pondered the fact that mostly women had been executed.

"How many?" a boy asked.

The girl who had been researching the play replied, "Fourteen women in Salem, more than a dozen more died in jail. Over history? Nobody knows for sure, certainly tens of thousands."

In Europe, most were burned at the stake because it was so painful, but sometimes they were hanged, drowned, or pressed to death with heavy boulders. Many of the women who were accused were older, displaced, or different in some way—easy targets.

"Mentally ill," I found myself whispering aloud with nothing to substantiate my comment, although what came to mind were images of my grandmother wandering in the pouring rain.

"Is that true? Were they mentally ill?" somebody asked.

"Maybe like the homeless in New York," someone added.

"A lot of them are Vets . . ."

The conversation continued and I thought about my brother's babblings and poetry, which had been so often religiously obsessed and fearful of possession. The patients in the Veterans' Hospitals had each seemed caught in some strange world and completely dependent on their caretakers. I swallowed thoughts of sleepwalking with a swig of beer. I'd felt myself disappearing before my classmates' eyes— quite the sorcerer's trick—and wrangled my mind back to the glass in my hand, to the feel of the wooden booth beneath my legs.

The conversation had turned to *One Flew Over the Cuckoo's Nest*, which was playing at the Thalia—a theatre devoted to showing classics and art films on the Upper West Side. Theo Mitsotakis, who'd been sitting next to me, leaned in close and asked me to join him for the late show. We'd had one date, but I didn't want any entanglements on the heels of my separation. He and I were always talking shop, each enamored of the other's angst and talent. Theo fared from a mythologically fucked-up Greek family, which had set the stage for him to grow up to be a big-hearted man, a ruthless philanderer, and a fine, fine actor. I knew that night by the way he pressed his leg into mine that he hoped for another date.

I'd avoided *One Flew Over the Cuckoo's Nest* for years, knowing it was set in the locked ward of a psychiatric hospital. Theo knew that I was legally separated from my husband, and I blamed my hesitation to see the film solely on my vulnerable state. "I have to get home to bed, I lied," but when he wouldn't let up, saying almost as a dare that the acting was superb, I conceded. Art came first between us.

All the characters affected me but especially Billy Bibbitt because he reminded me of my brother. Bibbitt was this sensitive, stuttering kid who was totally controlled by a sadistic nurse. Just when I thought he was going to get out from under her big-fat-stinking thumb, she threatened to tell his mother that he'd had sex with a girl. I was shocked by his bloody suicide and surprised by how much I wanted Jack Nicholson's character, McMurphy, to kill Nurse Ratched. I practically jumped out of my seat and cheered as he tried to strangle her. His failure left me completely deflated. When they rolled him out on a gurney after lobotomizing him, I nearly fainted.

As the lights came up in the theatre, I was crying hard without a single thought of control. Theo alternately held me and wiped away my tears with his bare hands. He pushed the sweaty hair from my forehead and looked at me with eyes so dark they were nearly black. When I calmed some, he took my hand in his.

"It was just so sad," I said, my voice far away as if it belonged to a girl in the next row. I looked down, not being able to receive his attention one second more and wishing—and not wishing—he'd let go of my hand.

"I have a brother who is . . . unwell," I whispered.

That was all I could muster in my shaky state, and we sat quietly until the usher had to clean our row. Theo squeezed my hand, not in a weird way, just a little to let me know he was still there and that we had to go.

"I can't take the subway."

"You don't have to."

We walked the few blocks to his place on Seventy-seventh Street, off Amsterdam Avenue, that he shared with some actors. Theo made me a cup of tea and played "The Lark Ascending" by Ralph Vaughn Williams, which I had never heard. The opening violin is like a person's spirit rising up free. I cried again unabashedly and told him about Billy, and Michael, and the sleepwalking too. I talked all night and he listened with his whole body like the goddamn excellent actor he was. It was like those sweet nights in the Hoffmans' golf shop. If only I'd been able to share the truth about my illness with Michael, maybe I wouldn't have run. With Don, I'd told him everything but had shared nothing. With Theo, I was able, for the first time in my life, to share some of my feelings about my malady with another person. If only that catharsis could have relieved the episodes.

We began dating and, like most actors, he was interested in all things psychological yet simultaneously unfazed by them. Together we developed a new form of denial—my episodes became a fascinating symptom of my tortured artist's soul and a subject for study.

I wasn't concerned about abandoning Theo after he saw me in the throes of a nocturnal fit because I knew he'd be leaving first. He'd been accepted to Yale Drama School and would start in the fall. However, he had to vacate his apartment by the end of June. Where I'd been staying in Brooklyn was unsafe, and I couldn't wait to move. I'd been offered a room with another classmate on the Upper West Side, but not until September. So when he asked me to share a sublet for July and August by Riverside Park, I said yes.

My sublet with Theo was a walkup on the top floor of a brownstone, a glorified boarding house. Our room belonged to Fred Hanson, an actor who'd landed an enviable internship at Williamstown Theatre

Festival in Massachusetts. It was an authentic bachelor pad and reminded me of a basement converted into a rec room. The bare walls were cheaply paneled and the corners were stacked with books, magazines, a deflated basketball, and an assorted variety of useless junk.

We shared a kitchen and bath with several other strangers who came and went at all hours. The place reminded me of a song my dad sang when I was a kid about a man and his shadow, who climbed the stairs each midnight, never bothering to knock because no one was there. My housemates seemed so lonely.

I was terrified of trying to survive in Manhattan and worked three waitressing jobs that summer. My insomnia escalated in a house with so many strangers and did not mix well with all the waitressing shifts. I couldn't keep up and both feared and hoped to be fired.

One brutally hot day, I was relieved to reach my air-conditioned job at the Empire Diner in Chelsea. When I wilted through the door, my manager scoffed at me in a voice loud enough for everyone to hear, "I saw you walking here on the sunny side of the street. What were you thinking?" *You, idiot*—his tone implied. "Why didn't you cross to the shade?" I was humiliated and further proved my stupidity by my blank expression, no repartee from me.

I escaped to the ladies' room, leaned my weary head against the mirror, and broke down. I'd been running late to work, which was becoming a habit. Once dawn arrived and made it safe for me to sleep, I couldn't rouse myself. Despite the unforgiving sun, I'd been too strung out to even think of crossing to the shade. As I cried in the bathroom, I imagined my grandmother, lost on her own street in a downpour.

The year 1984 became the summer of tears and I feared I was having a nervous breakdown for real. Theo was ever patient even while I feared falling apart. He read me plays in bed to calm my nerves—Chekov, Sam Shepard, Lillian Hellman. In addition to being overwrought about my failed marriage, grief-stricken over Michael's death, and dead on my feet from work, I simultaneously loved and hated my boyfriend for getting into Yale. I was jealous even though my better self considered it driftwood. If his talent was so recognized, mine would be too one day, wouldn't it?

Exhaustion increased my odds of having episodes, as did a strange environment. Theo was kind, but even after a few months his relief of leaving for New Haven was palpable. We had no bed, only a mattress on the floor, and the evening before we were to go our separate ways I lay on it, once again unable to sleep. There was a summer's worth of exhaustion weighing me down and stringing me out. It was 3:00 a.m., cool and rainy. Packed boxes surrounded us. Theo was asleep beside me, warm and snoring slightly, endearingly. He smelled like a man and I recalled how I loved waking my dad up on Saturdays with his stinky morning breath and his warnings to beware his rough beard on my baby fingers. Theo's stubble grew in a minute.

I studied his sleeping face. He had olive skin, classic features, and curly, black hair. His body was squat and strong. Dark fur covered his forearms and chest. His lips were a luscious mauve color and his brow furrowed. I wondered what he dreamt. He held the shiny trim of the blue blanket between his thumb and forefinger and rubbed the satiny material while he slept. I remembered failed efforts to soothe myself that same way as a kid.

I would miss him, no doubt, and was grateful for his attention as I'd left my marriage. I didn't do any of it gracefully but at least I'd gotten out. Just beneath the surface of my relief stirred the disgrace of having failed. I was a shameful Catholic girl in the night. I raised myself up on one arm and reached for my pack of cigarettes from the wooden crate that served as a bed stand. I'd switched from Luckies to Virginia Slims and smiled as I thought of my new slogan, *You've come a long way, baby*. Ha! How far, really, with my guilt nipping at my heels?

Naked, I perched on the edge of the mattress and paused before striking the match, wondering when it was, exactly, that I'd lost my faith—when Billy took ill, although I hadn't known it. For years, I went through the motions of prayer at Mass, but deep down in my broken heart the door to all things holy had been slammed shut and barred tight.

I struck the match, held it to my sexy cigarette and, thinking about my faithlessness, wished I could have set myself on fire. In certain cultures around the world, I would have been burned alive for adultery. My thoughts returned to the conversation with my fellow actors about witchcraft. I'd known about the burnings and hangings but hadn't known that some accused witches were drowned or pressed to death with heavy boulders. The memory of my near-drowning at the age of three rose like so much water.

In another time, I might have been accused of sorcery on account of the sleepwalking. Only a witch flies, screaming, through the night while sound asleep. People often disdain what they don't understand. I disdained myself.

I French inhaled, smoldering in my self-made cloud. I hardly lit up during the day, but nightly I lost myself in a haze of smoke. I carried it with me like Charlie Brown's friend, Pig-Pen. My love affair with cigarettes was—well, like playing with fire. I could not quit, despite the history of breast cancer in my family, not so long as they helped me stave off sleep. Forget about my fear of falling asleep while smoking.

A big tear splashed onto my dirty, red-lacquered toenail as I took another drag from my deathstick and dug my heels into the moldy carpet. There was a noise in the hall—someone creaking up the stairs. A chill spread over my bare skin and I suddenly felt unsafe. We only had a flimsy latch lock on the door. I crossed the room to check on it, carrying my cloud of smoke along for modesty's sake.

After listening at the door for who knows how long, I made my way back to Theo and sat again on the mattress to study him further. My hands shook. They'd been doing that all summer. I was used to it after an episode but not while wide awake. I thought of Billy's hands trembling so much at times that his glass of bedtime milk spilled and how I would hold it for him and help him drink it. But I decided that he was sick, while I was weak. It had taken Don's help to get me out of Albany to theatre school and it had taken Theo's help to keep me out of New Jersey and in the city. Maybe my manager at the Empire Diner was right. I was a dumb girl who couldn't make a move on my own.

I decided in that moment that I would never again marry or even let myself get serious with a man and felt a sudden urge to push Theo off the mattress or at least to pinch him awake. Instead, I hid my face from *I don't know who* and cried. Just as quickly as I'd felt like hurting my sleeping boyfriend, I felt like clinging to him and acting out a drama worthy of his Greek ancestors.

Instead, I extinguished my deathstick directly onto the wooden crate and reclined on the mattress. The drop ceiling was water-stained with ghostly shapes that seemed to patiently wait for me to slip into sleep, and I recalled the faces that used to emerge from the patterned wallpaper of my bedroom when I was little. My legs twitched from so many waitressing shifts and my feet were swollen like a pregnant lady's.

I closed my eyes and jolted awake from an instant dream of falling off a sidewalk. I was afraid. I was afraid to fall. I was afraid to fall asleep. I fought my body's desire to drift off. I worried over where we drift off to and how come I crash landed from one world to the next. If falling asleep was like a little bit of death each night, why couldn't I accept it, like my snoring fling? I remembered how easily Michael had fallen asleep with all he walked with. Why couldn't I go gently into that good night?

The rain on the roof soothed me with its rhythm—steady and sure. My eyes closed despite my best efforts to blink them open. Mother Nature hypnotized me against my will. I could not stop myself from opening the door dressed in stars and stepping over the threshold into the land of sleep.

I dreamt of lying, naked, in a dark pit in the ground. A heavy stone rested on my heart, racing in protest. The boulder pressed me down into the muck. It could press the life out of me with its steady burden. I'd been accused of witchcraft. Let them crush me through the very earth itself and into the underworld, but I would not admit to guilt that wasn't mine. Neither would I cry out. I would not give them the satisfaction.

I gasped to catch my breath and woke myself with a start. Where was I? Flat on my back, but where? There was the pitch black night and the sour smell of my animal fear. My heart galloped away beneath the imagined weight of the heavy stone. But it was real. I felt it still. For what heinous crime was I being punished? Each awakening from an episode carried the panic of being chased and underneath that panic, the blame of what I had done. It was the secret dread tucked so far away I could not name it—had I hurt someone or worse . . . while sleepwalking in a state akin to an alcoholic's blackout? This time I didn't run. I was frozen with fear. The burden on my sternum moved. After what seemed forever, I found the courage to touch it.

Theo's hand was resting over my chest in a protective pose. It was that weight that had entered my dream and startled me awake. I was not being pressed to death. For once, I was relieved to taste the tears that streamed down my face. I grabbed his hand and kissed it. He stirred slightly and cooed with his eyes still closed, "Don't worry, my little crab apple of a spirit." Theo was talking in his sleep. Even as I came out of my night terror, I recognized his altered state for what it was.

"Crab apple of a spirit," I whispered to myself—what a silly, curious phrase. Before I knew it we were spooning, and Theo was fondling the silky trim of our blanket while snoring happily away again. I'd never been so easily distracted after an episode, and I understood in that instant the extent to which he'd helped me through my summer of tears.

The next day, Theo left for New Haven and I moved in with my classmate a few blocks away. He hadn't fulfilled his playboy reputation when we'd lived together, but our long-distance relation-ship soon collapsed when he left me for the daughter of a famous actor. When I discovered he'd strayed, I thrashed about, playing the part of the wounded lover—but his infidelity was a kind of relief. My intuition had been correct—I'd only been able to stand the intimacy for so long. Theo's shoulder to cry on had made the shame of my failed marriage somewhat more bearable. For that I would be forever grateful. But sharing my real feelings about the sleepwalking had turned into a failed experiment. Even two months under an actor's microscope had been too long. I vowed never to get that close to anyone again. I imagined myself stepping into a protective armor. But even knights removed their mail upon repose. Thus my defense entrapped me.

FÜR ELISE

I did well at Circle-in-the-Square and showed great promise until, eventually, my performance reputation turned hit or miss. I could not consistently access my feelings. My illness had caused a crack in my psyche, or maybe a crack in my psyche had caused my illness. Either way, the fissure ran as deep and as far back as when I took those first unconscious nocturnal steps. Days filled with nonstop performance classes left my concentration teetering like a toddler's in need of a nap. I knew I was tired but denied the toll.

It baffled me why sometimes my work was brilliant and other times, not so much. Nikos Psacharopoulos had used the "b" word to describe my acting in his scene study class. He was our toughest instructor, who also taught at Yale and ran the most prestigious summer theatre in the country, Williamstown Theatre Festival, where Fred Haney had interned. I was overjoyed at his praise, hoping to be chosen to join him in Massachusetts the following season. However, halfway through my next scene, he barked his infamous, "Stop! What do you think you're doing?" I was heartbroken when he didn't award me an internship. All of my teachers acknowledged my talent but were wary. My inconsistency was a red flag and they wouldn't risk their reputations by recommending me for professional parts. I had acted the role of Invisible Girl for so long that I was clueless how to stop it, on stage or off. Fatigue affected every aspect of my life including my ability to understand, let alone trust my creative instincts.

While still in school, I auditioned for the soap opera *Guiding Light*. I was called back and put on tape. Casting for the contracted, principal role narrowed to between me and another girl. I didn't get it. A few weeks later, the casting director, Betty Rae, left me a message on my answering service late one day for what would have been my first professional speaking role on the next day's taping. It was a small part, a "five and under," which meant five or fewer lines. Acting, like any other business, is about building relationships. I missed her message. I'd been catching up on sleep that afternoon and retrieved it too late—after business hours. They'd hired someone else. She never called again.

Claudette Colbert, who began her career on Broadway and won the Academy Award for *It Happened One Night*, came to speak to my class. She'd been enjoying a resurgence of her theatrical career, earning a Sarah Siddons Award at the age of seventy-seven in 1980 for her work in a play in Chicago. One of my fellow students asked her to what she attributed her long and successful career. She answered, "Three square meals every day and a good night's sleep." Ms. Colbert admonished us for abusing our instruments by eating poorly and keeping late hours. I felt ashamed, as if I should have been able to control my dread of going to sleep. The experts who had written the *Psychology Today* article prescribed tolerance but they hadn't touched on how responsible the sleepwalker feels. I inevitably felt at fault.

By this time, Billy had quit drinking, which had always exacerbated his mental illness and compromised the efficacy of his psychiatric medicines. The revolving door in and out of hospitals stopped. The doctors were able to regulate his meds and he took them as prescribed. He began volunteering, reading text books aloud to a blind student named Sue at Albany State. She said it was love at first listen. Some students had been taunting her guide dog earlier that day, but my brother calmed them both with his gentle narration. Gypsy put her head in his lap and fell asleep. Billy and Sue married and enjoyed days full of reading, listening to music, and quiet companionship.

Just as my brother's life was coming together, mine began falling apart.

My first living situation after Theo was a rented room hardly big enough to turn around in at the back of an apartment on West Eighty-First Street. One thing I'd taken away from the previous summer was the good sense of sleeping close to the floor. It eliminated the height of a regular bed and felt safer when it came to dashing about while sound asleep. My roommate, Laura Livingston, held the lease. As landlady, she took the more spacious front room. A tiny kitchen and bathroom separated us.

Laura called herself a TAP, a Texan American Princess. She was a smart and talented actress with silky, golden locks, a milky complexion, and a heart the size of her home state. She never left the apartment without makeup and pranced easily in stilettos. "I don't know how you can stand to walk in those heels," I said to her once. She sassed back, "Honey, I don't know how you can stand to walk without 'em!" Laura used old-fashioned body powder, the kind with a puff, and wore lady slippers decorated with similar pink puffs like Barbie's. She wore scarves and perfume and was forever trying to teach me her wily ways, but I thought her efforts a waste of time, preferring to repulse rather than attract any serious courters.

My roommate was a mystic. She introduced me to the I Ching and bought me my first deck of tarot cards. I had a knack for interpreting both, but their power seemed separate from my own. I anxiously searched for answers to deep and daft questions like the emotionally insecure child I was.

Laura nicknamed me Mookie, as in Mookie Wilson, well-loved outfielder and base-stealer from the Mets. He led that scrappy team. I guess she saw me as a bit of an underdog and, in our early friendship, as the little athlete of art that could. She was an empathetic soul, even while perplexed and sometimes horrified by my nocturnal handicap and its effects. If she'd been privy to an episode, next morning she'd let me know by humming "Walking After Midnight" as she two-stepped about the kitchen, making me a cup of tea to calm my nerves. I was reminded of my vigils on the Jersey streets in the middle of those interminable nights after Michael's death, listening to Patsy Kline over and over again on my Walkman.

At this juncture, I began waking more frequently during sleep-walking. More often than not, I'd forget about it come morning. Some-times I'd drop it completely from my memory. Other times, flashes of my wandering would startle me from my day. I'd heard that women forget the pain of childbirth in order to be able to have another baby. I wondered if my amnesia was similar, although my oblivion never seemed to ease my terror of the night. Then there were the incidents of total recall, detailed and eerie like an Edgar Allan Poe tale.

It was as dark as a movie theater and I seemed to be both in the film and watching myself wander someplace. I felt lost in the woods only without the trees. My hands groped at the air as if I were blind. I panicked and reached for anything familiar. I grabbed at the walls for safety's sake but they'd disappeared. I freaked. Where was I? Was I emerging from an episode? I was turning in frantic circles as classical music played. My mind gripped to name the piece but to no avail. A gown brushed against my legs as I spun but it could have been my long, flannel nightgown.

I smelled something sweet and realized that in my hand was an Easter bun with raisins and two strips of icing across the sticky, golden top—a hot cross bun made by my paternal grandmother. Images flew by, as if I was spinning through time, like Dorothy tossed by the tornado on her way to Oz. There was Grandma Frazier's long face with the mole on her chin and a hair growing out of it. Her blue eyes were sad, and just as we'd reached out our hands to touch each other, the vortex had drawn us apart. I wished I could have felt her soft, white hair, pulled up into a bun, sweet like the sugar bun that had disappeared from my turning hand, an offering to no one there.

I saw my other grandma, Grandma Tallmadge, holding a baby, and I knew it was me bundled in her arms from the story my mother would tell of how happy she'd been to have held me as an infant—just before she died. Then Billy's face flew by, and Michael's too. I was losing everyone along the way and I began to cry. I had become a stringed puppet girl. Someone laughed manically from above but I could not see his face.

Thump. I landed like the house upon the Wicked Witch.

Was I back in my sweating body, bumping toward consciousness? I found myself flat-out on my futon, or so I surmised from the scratch of my woolen blanket—my candy blanket from Grandma Frazier—bunched in my fists. I pulled it to my chin. It was winter but the radiator had broken in my rear room and spewed steam. Despite the heat, I'd gone from perspiring to shivering in the moments it took to place myself. A siren echoed from the street, round the alley, up five flights, and through my open window—a lonely, city sound. My cheeks were wet with emotion from dreaming about my grannies, my brother, and Michael. Aside from the sleep tears, it seemed like a nightmare—only a nightmare, thank goodness, like regular people got. Maybe. I wiped away my tears with the soft sleeve of my nightdress.

Icy rain pelted garbage cans below and the radio alarm clock read 1:00 a.m. Suddenly, "Fur Elise" blasted from Piano Boy—my neighbor boy across the alley who played the piano. He was manic and would burst into music anytime of the day or night. I wondered if he'd been playing while I'd slept, if his tune had turned me into a whirling dervish in my dream. I continued to worry if it had only been a nightmare. I glanced around and no objects had been knocked over. Still, there was no definitive way of knowing if I'd danced around my room while sound asleep.

The young musician could both enthrall and torture with his gift. He often broke down into fits of laughter or fits of tears over the keys.

Maybe he'd been my hysterical puppeteer. He was a child prodigy, out of control the night of my spinning dream. God, how he banged away. "Shut it!" called a neighbor from his window but he did not get a response. I'd have closed my own but for the heat. My chills subsided as my anger rose.

I threw off the candy blanket with its dead memories weighing me down. I was sweating again and felt trapped in my tiny time capsule of a room. How do astronauts keep from going mad, I wondered? Regan came to mind, how she predicted the astronaut's death in *The Exorcist*. My skin crawled as if covered with ants everywhere, every single place. I wanted to hit myself in the head and pull out my hair. I craved escape but had hardly slept.

Fear of the dark descended fully then, but I didn't want to turn on the overhead light. The bare bulb offended me and simple tasks like buying a shade or replacing the radiator cap felt overwhelming. The smell of sulphur filled the air as I struck a wooden match against its box. I lit my favorite candle—a flicker of safety in the night. It was red and smelled rosy, and the holder was fashioned like a stain glassed window with a rose on it. My mother's name was Catherine Rose, and even though I was a full grown woman and she was miles away in Albany, I missed her.

I hummed a lullaby to myself in my hot little room accompanied by the hissing radiator but had no luck. Piano Boy drowned me out. Surrendering to his superior talent and with candle in hand—like an old-fashioned girl—I ventured to the window and knelt on the hardwood floor to listen. Beethoven burned through the centuries. My chest ached for something I couldn't put my finger on.

Images of the Sacred Heart came to mind, so often depicted with his illuminating flame. I'd recently discovered St. Malachy's, the actors' chapel on Forty-Ninth Street. I'd no desire to return to the fold, but took great comfort in lighting a votive and praying before a magnificently tiled image of Christ pointing to his fiery heart as if to say, *here's the answer—look inside.* I'd kneel in front of that mosaic and pray gratitude for Billy's returning health, and for my mother's.

She was in remission. I'd whisper my desire to keep my heart in my work and always, always, begged for rest.

The boy's playing turned exquisitely sotto and I thought about my most recent flame, Theo, playing "The Lark Ascending" to calm me down when we'd first met and how I couldn't seem to let men love me for very long.

Just as suddenly, the music turned raucous again. "Shut the hell up!" boomed another man's voice from below, but I'd begun to figure Piano Boy for a kindred spirit on that sleepless night. I leaned on the windowsill, craning my neck to look out. His silhouette looked like a shadow puppet through the lacy curtains. Cool rain fell upon my face. If only it could baptize me, but I felt beyond redemption.

Piano Boy's mother began hollering at him in response to the second man's complaint. Her voice was repulsive, like the Sea Hag from Popeye. He played faster and louder and I reached for an unopened package of cigarettes. The fresh plastic wrapper was smooth and cool. I loved the way they smelled but didn't dawdle. I lit one and, leaning out the window again, blew rings of smoke over to the boy. Smoke signals, DON'T . . . GIVE . . . UP.

She slapped him then across the back of his head and the music stopped. I felt weirdly responsible. Sometimes he wouldn't stop when it came to blows. Sometimes he played more furiously. This was their pattern, like a sickness between them. But that night he closed the lid, buried his head in his arms, and sobbed over his shut up instrument.

I pretended they weren't real, that I had dreamt them. My chest heaved but I was too tired to cry. I felt like a sack of potatoes; I felt like something that got dragged around a while. I wanted to save that boy from his screaming mother. I concentrated on French inhaling my cigarette and took pleasure from the burning in my nose and throat, punishment for my powerlessness over everything that seemed to matter in life.

I had to escape the boy and his mother. I would leave. My room-mate's steady boyfriend was staying over, and I decided to risk the awkwardness of running into one of them in our cramped quarters. I tore off my granny gown and pulled on my ripped jeans with holes in the knees, and threw on a T-shirt and jacket. I hardly had my wits about me, sleep deprived as I was, but instinctively grabbed my long-handled purse that I wore across my chest to lessen my chances of being mugged. Thieves looked for vulnerable victims on the darkened streets of Manhattan. I tossed my package of Marlboros in there. I'd dropped Virginia Slims when I'd dropped all pretense of being a lady.

I tiptoed through the apartment and paused to put on my boots in the kitchen, which led to the building's hallway. Laughter and light slipped from where Laura's closed door didn't meet the floor. She loved entertaining and I felt waves of jealousy and nausea.

Outside, the air woke me completely. We'd had a beautiful snowstorm the previous week but the streets had turned filthy with brown banks and huge puddles at the corners. The sidewalks were heavily salted in front of the buildings with conscientious supers and thick with ice where others had been lazy. I stepped gingerly, fearful as I was of falling in my exhausted state. I finished my cigarette, threw down the butt, and stepped on it—pretended it was Piano Boy's mother and squashed it good. It was satisfying to crush it to smithereens. The temperature was on the rise and had turned the precipitation into a light mist. I closed my umbrella and turned my face upward. I opened my hands to catch the raining kisses. My rising mood was dashed when a couple of turtledoves cooed past me arm in arm, laughing their secret laugh.

I slowly slipped and slid over to Marvin's Garden on Broadway. *I don't need a boyfriend.* I tried to convince myself when I was about to savor the restaurant's signature dessert—chocolate, chocolate chip cake with homemade whipped cream. I would order a slice to go, devour it alone in my room, and pass out from the sugar rush.

Laughter from the bar reminded me of *Cheers,* only unlike that show's theme song, nobody knew my name since the establishment was expensive for me. The bartender asked me if I'd like a drink while

I waited for my order but I refused. I was on the wagon. I'd begun to worry over my sensitivity to the stuff. I sometimes forgot the events of an evening after a single drink and absolutely hated losing control. It was too much like sleepwalking.

I Love Lucy played on a television hung overhead. Some people laughed but others just drank. They didn't pretend to be social. Lucy wallpapered Ethel to the wall. As a kid, I'd yelled at Lucy to stop it, just stop it—don't do the obviously stupid thing—but she never listened. It's why people loved Lucy, but I did not love Lucy.

However romantic the rain had been on my outbound trip, the weather had turned nasty, my flimsy umbrella flew inside out, and I arrived home wet and shivering. Laura's room was quiet but a roach welcomed me, scurrying across the kitchen floor in the light from the building's hallway. I stomped it and our downstairs insomniac neighbor pounded her ceiling with the broom she kept ready. It was going on 2:00 a.m. My face turned red for no one to see.

I snuck into my room, cake bag in hand. I'd left the candle burning. My heart beat, *stupid-girl, stupid-girl* and any trace of common sense wagged its frantic finger in my face. I'd forgotten to snuff it out on account of my fatigue. Fuck it. It was safe inside the holder, I lied to myself.

My damp jeans stuck to me but I disrobed as fast as I could. I hoped they'd packed a fork but would have eaten it by the fistful rather than risk, for a second time, the chance of running into Laura or what's his name. The cake beckoned through the plastic take-out container. The bottom was aluminum and I hated its taste but quieted my inner snob with the thought, *Let them eat cake on aluminum.* Hallelujah, I'd found the plastic fork. The first bite dispelled all concerns over my fat thighs and was almost too much to bear. I sat on the futon and consumed the cake, naked, by candlelight.

Afterward, somebody turned on a light in an apartment in the adjacent building, and it reflected through my solitary window directly onto my lap. It seemed to dance, a Tinkerbell fairy. I put down the empty take-out pan and caught the magical creature in my bowled hands. I drank it. I swallowed it whole in hopes of rekindling my own diminishing light. But that flicker made me sick to my stomach, or maybe it was the cake. I placed my hand on the top of my head where the bone is thick, no escape. I hated being human with no one dear and near to clap my spirit awake.

I lay down on the futon and pulled my sheets about me. They were from my childhood, patterned with pastel, faded stripes. I felt a heaviness in my arms and legs and in my chest. My eyelids drooped. The candle shone red through the rose glass holder. I knew I should snuff it out but couldn't bear the thought. I just had to leave that little light on. With the candle going, I might come back into my body faster after a night terror or if I sleepwalked.

Suddenly I felt panicked, on the run, on the lamb, and listed my fears to me, myself, and I—noisy boys, jarring sounds, someone coming to get me, someone trying to kill me, nuclear holocaust, death by fire, death by suffocation, drowning by loneliness, dying in my sleep. I was afraid of falling asleep, of not falling asleep, of falling down, of being seen, of not being seen, of being paralyzed. And that's what happens when you sleep. You're paralyzed. Unless you're not. Unless you walked, like me.

There used to be an old man who lived in the apartment next to ours. Laura and I would see him occasionally, drunk in the dark bars of Hell's Kitchen—Morahan's, Film Center Café, or Rudy's. Then his dream came true: he retired. His drinking picked up. We'd have to step over him when he passed out, shoeless on the stoop or in the hallway with his pants pissed or worse. Then we didn't see him for some time, but our cockroach problem grew. A sickeningly sweet smell permeated the hallway outside his apartment. The police were called and entered his place through our shared fire escape.

Laura and I weren't told much until the uniforms called the detectives and they called us in to identify the body. I'd only seen

Grandma Frazier lying in state in a funeral parlor when I was seven, but this old man was not surrounded by flowers nor had anyone tenderly arranged a rosary in his folded hands. He was prone, face up on a dirty, single daybed with dried blood caking the pillow. The mirror in his nearby bathroom was cracked and a trail of blood led from there to where he lay. The cops surmised that he'd fallen while drunk into the bathroom mirror, which caused a deep gash in his forehead. Oblivious to his fatal wound, he lay down and bled to death. He bumped his head, he went to bed, and he didn't get up in the morning.

All at once I felt weighty with sleep despite my gruesome bedtime story. The sugary cake had done its duty. Sometimes, when I was between the worlds of asleep and awake, I imagined myself floating above myself in my room. This night, my body was tense, my hands in fists, my shoulders by my ears, my brow furrowed. It's a wonder I ever fell asleep at all. I felt sad for my body down there. If only I could have held myself like Mary held Jesus in the statue of the Pieta. I would have whispered lovingly but emphatically into my nearly sleeping ear, DON'T . . . GIVE . . . UP. Shadows wavered from the little candle in the wind, but it didn't blow out.

The next thing I remembered was the feeling of running. I didn't know if I was dreaming or awake until I slipped and would have fallen except my hands slapped and grabbed onto something hard and cold, something familiar. It seemed that I'd landed upon a sink and it startled me back into my body. It was like trying to fit a camel through the eye of a needle, fast. My heart beat crazily and sweat spilled down my cheeks, or were they tears?

I'd been running away from whatever was coming to get me. I was not convinced of my whereabouts. Was it really a sink I gripped? Was it my bathroom sink or that of my dead, drunk neighbor's? I was standing, shivering in the dark somewhere, holding on for dear life. The smell of flowery perfume clued me in—I was in my own apartment bathroom. The feminine scents lingered where Laura had prepared for her date. I felt for the light switch and flicked it. I'd forgotten I was naked and closed and locked the door. I leaned against it and a roach scurried alongside the baseboard. I worried that it might have been a roach that had startled me into a terror. I despised the necessity of sleeping on a futon and feared my close proximity to the filthy creatures. Or maybe Piano Boy had started up again but his Sea Hag mother had put a stop to it just as quickly. I didn't know. I almost never knew what brought on an episode no matter how painstakingly I searched my mind, no matter how frantically I rifled through my dreams.

I fought to catch my breath, to escape from the land of the living dead. *Look about, come to*, I pressed myself. The floor was covered with a fine dusting of Laura's body powder, which is how I'd slipped and fallen onto the sink. I stepped away from the door and faced the mirror. I dug my fingers into the basin. I clawed my way back into this world. I splashed cold water over my face and convinced myself that it wasn't so bad this time. No, not too bad. I hadn't screamed or woken up my roommate or her boyfriend. I didn't want to bother anybody. I stared at myself in the mirror above the sink and said aloud, "I didn't. I didn't bump my head and go to bed and didn't get up in the morning."

I sidestepped the sink and rested my cheek against the cold glass, relieved that the episode was over.

All of a sudden, I was struck sleepy. I could have fallen out, leaning there against the hard, cold porcelain. I wrapped myself in a towel and led myself back to my room, alive and calm at last. I barely made it to the futon before dropping to my knees as if I'd been shot in the back like in an old western. I fell on the futon, into it, through it. I sunk into the deepest, sorely earned sleep with the little candle light still flickering beside me in the night.

LOOKING FOR
MR. GOODBAR

Not long after the night of Fur Elise, Laura announced she wanted the place to herself. I was too ashamed to ask if somnambulism played a part in my eviction. I didn't blame her. Leaving candles to burn while one slept, let alone while making a cake run, was a capital offense in any apartment mate's book and reasonably punishable by exile.

I took another tiny room in a rambling apartment on West End and 101st Street with four partiers from my school. Maybe my somnambulism would go unnoticed alongside their carousing. I found myself joining in as a way to further camouflage my illness. People did a lot of things while under the influence that were like night terrors and sleepwalking. And the effects of my worsening insomnia were similar to symptoms of a hangover—fatigue, headache, sensitivity to light and noise, body aches, and tremors.

In 1983, we finished the program at Circle-in-the-Square and had a showcase for industry professionals. A few agents interviewed me, we agreed to freelance, and they sent me out on the occasional audition, but I lacked energy to follow up. Many successful actors attribute their good fortune to suiting up and showing up—99 percent perspiration and 1 percent inspiration. I was all too eager to work and my gift was apparent, but sleepwalking, night terrors, and the ensuing insomnia rendered me incapable of the required discipline. Those in the position to hire smelled my insecurity as surely as a predator smells the weakest prey.

I kept up my craft by taking Saturday classes with my favorite teachers, Terese Hayden and Jacqueline Brooks, from The Actors Studio. Over the next year, they convinced me to audition for those hallowed halls of acting fame. I fashioned a scene from Salinger's *Franny and Zooey* in which I played Franny Glass, a girl in her twenties smack in the middle of a nervous breakdown or existential crisis, depending on how you looked at it. Her brother, Seymour, had served in World War II, returned home traumatized, and committed suicide. Franny couldn't accept that time marched on after her brother's suffering. Her college classmates seemed petty and her studies trivial in the face of her loss. She was wan from insomnia. During the course of the passage, Zooey, her other brother, persuades her to not give up.

My scene partner and I were called back to repeat our work in the final auditions in June, 1984. Maybe it was because I'd hardly any acting to do for the part that my work earned me a place as a finalist for the 1984–85 season. It was quite an honor and enabled me to attend the twice weekly acting sessions to observe talented members' work and hear critiques by Elia Kazan, Harvey Keitel, and Ellen Burstyn, to name a few. I also could have worked in a scene during the session with a member, but was too shaky to approach anyone. During this year of privileges, I was supposed to be preparing for my final audition. Instead I slept my days away and made every effort to stay up nightly. And I drank. I was a terrible drinker but kept at it with a vengeance. Far from easing the somnambulism, it further compromised my health.

My ability to function, or lack thereof, was marked by my waitressing gigs on the Upper West Side. First, I created Caesar salad and steak tartare tableside at Prime Time, a high-class steak house. One night, I served a friend of Don's parents who ridiculed me about the synonymy of "actress and waitress." His table of fat businessmen laughed derisively. It was like he'd stuck his porky finger in my soft underbelly and, upon extraction, out flopped my failed marriage and faltering career all over the serving tray. I was too tired to do anything but burst into tears. The kindly waitstaff ushered me to the ladies' room and took over the table.

Then I worked at Copper Hatch II, more of a middle-class place owned by the same restaurateurs. More often than not, I joined my coworkers after shifts to party the night away or to pretend to party the night away. If I could just get to morning, I could rest. My pattern of never having a somnambulant episode during the day continued.

By twenty-four, I ended up as a barmaid at P&G's, a dive on Seventy-Second Street. The neon sign outside had a flashing martini glass nestled between the words STEAKS, CHOPS. It looked like the bad bar in *It's a Wonderful Life* when George Bailey sees what the world would be like without him—a nice family tavern distorted into a sleazy, smoke-filled gin mill. P&G patrons were mostly older men who drank to get plastered. They made me their mascot. I became one of the boys and matched them drink for drink. By last call, the place was littered with angry drunks fetching for a fight. Like me, nobody wanted to go home.

I grew afraid for future me as I doggedly raised my glass and annihilated my feelings. My drinking buddies offered a warning, like the Ghost of Christmas Future in Dickens's cautionary tale. Only I was unable to open my weary eyes long enough to take heed.

There were always people who cared for me, including several fellows I dated. Problem was their attention repulsed me. I'd go out of my way to avoid sleeping with them. If a man so much as hinted at further attachment, I'd break it off before he could realize how sick I was and leave me.

I grew desperately lonely and began picking up guys in bars rather than face the abyss of bed alone. I'd come to Manhattan, hoping for a life in the theatre. What I got was a run of sleepwalking performances, sometimes with a shocked audience, sometimes solo. Just like in college, I chose promiscuity in an effort to both have a bed partner and avoid the intimacy of a long-term relationship. Danger heightened in a city that was burgeoning with AIDS. I put myself in many life-threatening situations from unprotected sex to slapping strangers in Hell's Kitchen. I became completely out of control and often didn't know whether I was waking from a blackout or from a violent sleepwalking episode.

I suddenly found myself splayed out on an icy sidewalk on a darkened side street of what appeared to be my neighborhood but really could have been any number of places. The fading bulb of a nearby streetlamp shed meager light. Disheveled brownstones loomed and bare trees shivered in the blustery wind. I was flat on my back and leaned up on one elbow. Where the hell was I?

It was a bitter winter night, no traffic or people to be seen. Panic overtook me. My last memory had been a warm barroom filled with raucous laughter, the result of one of my witticisms. Had I nodded off and fallen off the stool like once before, only to be shown the door? Was I slumbering still, with the deserted city street the hallucinated scene of this night's terror?

It seemed I was able to materialize and dematerialize—only, sadly, not at will. My heart sank with shame. I felt as though I were disappearing before my very eyes. *Kathy's so quiet, you wouldn't even know she was here.* Maybe all that play at being invisible as a kid had finally taken hold. I was the Invisible Woman.

The freezing sidewalk seemed solid enough beneath my bare hands. I managed to sit up. My new red cowboy boots were already ruined from salt, but at least they were on my feet. Once, I'd come to propped against my apartment building holding a single shoe, reminiscent of my poor neighbor at Laura's place. I checked for my purse, intact across my chest.

The wind blasted my face, and with it a plastic bag spooked me from a nearby garbage can that'd blown its lid. I swatted the trash away and pulled close my navy blue, cashmere car-coat that I'd purchased secondhand at Alice's Underground for only seven dollars. It was my pride and joy, however threadbare, and the wind blew right through it. The wind blew through my mini skirt, and black tights, black silk turtleneck, which smelled of body odor but I was too lazy to wash by hand. The wind blew through my bones and rattled my intoxicated heart 'round my ribcage. And the wind blew through my long, curly, brown hair, picking it straight up and all about my head like a nest to comfort my fluttering eyes, twin birds set in my frozen face. My face felt numb. I was a numbskull. I saw myself clearly on the darkened street, same as between the worlds of asleep and awake, when I'd leave my body to gaze at myself below. Maybe I was dead, and I read the headlines in my mind, BEAUTIFUL DEAD-DRUNK GIRL FOUND WITH FROZEN FACE.

Everything sunk hopelessly, but despite my animal fear of the situation in which I'd found myself, I was unable to stand and leave it. I crawled on all fours and sat on the edge of the curb but couldn't right myself completely. I searched for a street sign but had landed in the middle of a block. If I could just have one more martini straight up with extra olives, I knew I would have found the strength to set sail for home, slip-sliding as I'd go.

The warmth of tears surprised me as they made effort to defrost my icy countenance. I was amazed at how hotly they poured forth on that frigid night. I wiped my eyes, smearing my mascara across the back of my hand and thought—there goes my false face. I dropped my head across my arms and cried wholeheartedly at the loss.

My sobs were broken by the sound of footsteps behind me. I was not alone and got a terrible feeling that someone had been watching me. That woke me up.

Beside me appeared two men's black leather boots and a pair of well-cut black woolen trousers. European, I guessed. I became certain as I continued gazing upward, taking inventory. But was he phantom or real? If imagined, his imaginary overcoat was beautifully tailored, black also. Even make-believe American men didn't know how to dress this well. He reminded me of Italians I'd met when I toured with the youth theatre. He seemed awfully real for a ghost. Everything about him was dark—olive skin, dark eyes, and curly brown hair. Backlit by the dim streetlamp, he looked like a haloed saint in a Renaissance fresco. My heart raced. Did I know him? Had I invited him home from the pub? He gazed on me with heavenly pity and extended one hand with long fine fingers to help me stand.

The moment we touched, all the baby hairs on the nape of my neck bristled and something inside of me screamed no. But I was miles from listening to my intuition and unsteady on my feet. He clucked his tongue, "Bella, Bella, are you all right? No, of course not."

He was Italian or pretended to be. We stood face-to-face. His breath was warm and sweet from some syrupy liqueur. He steadied me on my feet and, in a gesture of familiarity, brushed dirty ice from the bottom of my coat with his free hand. One minute I felt repulsed by his intimate advances and the next I wanted to slip beneath his open coat, which he could have easily wrapped around me.

"I pass you coming up the street in the taxi and I tell the driver let me out up the square, I mean, the block. You had fallen on this, how you say, icy and I see you needed help."

He seemed tailor-made for me in his tailored clothes. If we'd met at the bar, I'd have scooped him up like so much spumoni and brought him home for dessert, but it dawned on me that I'd seen no cab pass by. Maybe I'd been passed out or sleeping. I realized that he was still holding my hand and I felt both butterflies and sick to my stomach. I stepped back but he didn't let go.

"No, thank you. No help needed. I'm fine," even as I nearly faltered again.

"Miss Bella. I think maybe too much . . ." and he mimed the universal sign for drinking.

I shook my head no, smiled, and shuffled nervously. My hand went limp in his, like a fish, and began flopping its way loose of his grip. Reluctantly, he released me.

"Please, maybe I should walk you home?"

Wow, how nice that would be if only I could be certain that you aren't a serial killer, I thought, and *Looking for Mr. Goodbar* flashed through my mind. Not the horrific murder scene but earlier that same night when the mild-mannered schoolteacher by day confides to the bartender that it will be her last night of wandering—ha, nocturnal wandering. He declines her offer of a drink, explaining, "Between you and me, one is too many and a thousand is never enough." She quips, "Yeah, that's how it is with me and men."

"Please Miss Bella, I mean you no . . . how you say . . . harm." And in a gesture of innocence, he stood before me and opened his arms wide. His unbuttoned coat billowed, a villain's cape in the wind, and I glimpsed a knife attached to his belt, not a Swiss Army knife but a hunting one, secured in a leather sheath. The hair on my forearms stood to attention, an army of soldiers set for the fight, as he smiled and I realized that he'd intended for me to see the weapon. He knew I could neither run nor fight on that empty, slippery street in my condition.

I inhaled, a singer's breath, to scream awake the neighborhood, but then my throat restricted, like in the recurring nightmare of drowning I'd had since before the sleepwalking. He laughed at my impotence and grabbed my arm—hard. At the same moment, a light came on outside the door of the nearest brownstone and an old man grumbled out. He had a puppy tucked under one arm, like a football, and was climbing into an overcoat with the other. My assailant pushed me down and ran away. The dog barked and my rescuer climbed down the steps to my aid.

He helped me up and I held out my hands to see them shaking, just like after a violent somnambulant episode. I still couldn't speak, and for a split second I wondered if I had dreamt the whole ordeal— was dreaming still if it weren't for the man in his pajamas and winter coat standing before me in the flesh with his German Shepard puppy barking away. My mind gripped on the fact of the dog's breed and how Michael's had been so loyal.

"Loyal, so loyal," I babbled aloud.

The stranger was patting my back and puffs of steam escaped his mouth, but I had no idea what he was saying. He repeated something over and over, trying desperately to calm me. Finally his words came clear, "You're all right. You're going to be all right." I nodded my head, double time, but it was only to appease that kind gentleman who'd saved my life. I knew I was as far from all right as a young woman could possibly get.

THE LOST AND FOUND
WEEKEND

I 've heard that addiction is the thing we do so that we do not have to face the thing that scares us. I've also heard that a periodic is a scared daily drinker, and that's what I became on the heels of my near-death experience. I'd abstain completely for weeks on end until the anticipation of sleepwalking, the shame of an episode, and/or the stress of exhaustion dictated release. Just as I tolerated the somnambulism, I tolerated the consequences of my release.

Final auditions for The Actors Studio occurred again in June 1985. I'd fashioned a scene from Hemmingway's *For Whom The Bell Tolls*, as I'd done with Salinger's *Franny and Zooey* for the previous year. The story takes place during the Spanish Civil War in the midst of guerilla warfare. I played Maria, a shattered girl of nineteen who'd been raped by the fascists and traumatized by her parents' executions. She and Robert Jordan, an American dynamite expert, had fallen in love. The passage takes place during their final moments together, after Jordan is wounded and will not escape death at the hands of the enemy. His comrades must leave him behind. Maria cannot bear to abandon him, but he convinces her that she must go, survive, and carry on for the both of them.

In real life, I'd never been able to shake my guilt over leaving Michael to face death alone and denied the role my somnambulism had played in my fear of intimacy. In real life, I minimized the deadly circumstances in which I placed myself on account of my blackout drinking. But the artist in me was not so ignorant. I begged my own attention in choosing the life or death scene.

I hadn't had a drink for days before my audition but neither had I slept. I was strung out and fatigued to the point of collapse. I froze up and hid from the audience of judges by standing behind my scene partner. I'd lost my ability to be vulnerable on stage, having so long considered it a weakness in life. The failed audition proved that my armor of indifference was not so easily removed at will. I could not lay down my shield when I stepped on stage and pick it up again when the work ended. My defenses had become fixed.

The following Saturday, I slumped into Terry Hayden and Jackie Brooks's class and was promptly called out. They had heard about my debacle at the Studio. Terry ordered me to sit alone on a folding chair on the stage, facing my fellow actors. She stared me down. My lip quivered but she never wavered. "When are you going to take responsibility for your talent?"

Her words hung in the air. A death sentence. Only I held the power to order a stay of execution.

"There's always next year," I sassed softly even as my eyes filled with tears.

"This is no game," she warned. "Fuck the Studio. I'm talking about your life."

I broke down.

"Don't you dare romanticize this!"

Terry knew me well enough from class, and we sometimes lunched as a group afterward. I'd been glamorizing the tragic demise of Studio giants like James Dean, Montgomery Clift, and Marilyn Monroe. She'd seen plenty of actors fall prey to the addictions that destroyed first their gifts and then their lives. I figured I wouldn't live beyond the age of twenty-five and my twenty-sixth birthday was only a few months away. I could not stand much more. In those moments, as I trembled in the spotlight of my teacher's attention, some part of me understood that I would not be able to stand much more. Images of my brother's bandaged wrists filled my head, but I could not peep a word.

My teacher didn't know the cause of my suffering but her tough love had landed my heart—an expertly placed arrow through a chink in my armor.

The first week of July, the official letter arrived from The Actors Studio. It confirmed that I had not been selected for membership or even for an additional year as a finalist with privileges. If I dared further interest, I could start from scratch with another preliminary audition the following season.

The fourth of July fell on a Thursday. I waitressed that evening at P&G's. After my shift, the bartender offered me one on the house. I gave in. That's the last I remember until I came to, awakened by my own piercing screams.

A giant prehistoric bird, a pterosaur, was diving straight for me. The gapping jaw displayed rows of razor-sharp teeth, poised for the kill. It wildly flapped huge, bat-like wings and glared with beady yellow eyes, with jagged talons outstretched. Claws dug deep into the flesh of my unprotected forearms. Shrieking madly, I scratched at my arms in an effort to dislodge the bird. It tightened its grip. I writhed frantically, tearing at my own skin.

Then I saw the terrified face of an old cabby staring back at me from his front seat like a frame frozen in a film. I was in the backseat of a cab. The prehistoric bird disappeared as suddenly as it had appeared but, for a moment, I continued to shriek, dig at my arms, and flail at the empty air.

The driver gasped in horror, pulled over to the sidewalk, and motioned for me to get the hell out. I couldn't seem to budge, shocked as I was that the object of this evening's terror had stalked me to this extent. The driver was hollering now, but I couldn't distinguish his words; I could only see his mouth moving. Looking down, the skin on my forearms was bleeding, really bleeding, from where I had clawed away my own flesh to free myself from the imagined pterosaur. I opened the door and practically rolled out of the car into the city night. I landed on wet pavement into a full-fledged summer thunderstorm.

I awoke dressed in my waitressing uniform, face down on my futon. Eventually, I figured that it was early evening—Friday, July 5—but I was unaware of how I'd gotten home or if I was alone. My roommates were supposed to be away that holiday weekend. I searched the apartment, steak knife in hand. After the night of Looking for Mr. Goodbar, I'd slept with the weapon at my side. How easily I could have turned it against one of my unsuspecting roommates during a somnambulant episode or a blackout, mistaking them for an assailant. How easily I could have turned it against myself.

The place was empty. Even so, I sat in my room with the door locked and tried to soothe myself by rocking in the rocking chair that Mary Ann had given me when I'd gone off to college. The mirror on the back of my door reflected a ghostly girl. My face was bloated from boozing and my hair was turning prematurely gray. Early silvers ran in my family, but I guessed the continuous frights also had something to do with it.

I held the knife in my lap for a long time, trying to piece together the puzzle of the previous night. Most parts had vanished. More terrifying than any horror movie was *The Lost Weekend*. In it, Ray Milland loses a whole weekend in a blackout. It had been my parents' first date, a foreshadowing of my father's alcoholism. But it was not *my* story. I wasn't a middle-aged man like my dad had been when he'd bottomed out, or Ray Milland's character, or the patrons at P&G's.

I searched and searched my memory. Only the harrowing hallucination in the cab came back clearly, too clearly. Why couldn't I have conjured a friendly pooka, like Jimmy Stewart's six-foot rabbit in

Harvey? I shuddered at the thought of being eaten alive by my own imagination. I shivered at the thought of being lost in the drenching rain, which had been quite real. Grandma Tallmadge came to mind and I wondered if it had finally happened. I'd cracked beyond repair. I feared being institutionalized. I dreaded shock treatments most of all. Euthanasia was more humane and I wished for a friend to help put me out of my misery. The rusty kitchen knife was a dull companion.

I stole a razor blade from my apartment mate's room and tucked it beneath my pillow for safe keeping.

I called in sick to work that night. Anyone could see I was ill, besides being petrified to leave the apartment. To make matters worse, it was July 5, the day Don and I married and what would have been our fifth anniversary.

I needed courage for what I contemplated and located a bottle of cheap champagne that I'd hidden from myself in the back of my closet. Some date had left it behind after storming off when I'd told him that we were through. I worried that drinking alone would make me an alcoholic and hated the idea of being discovered with an empty bottle by my side. I was a people pleaser even as I planned my own demise. I thought to go out for a quick one, just one, but decided to face the night's terror alone. I'd rather be my own undoing than be undone by Mr. Goodbar.

After my first coffee mug of champagne, I decided to honor my last request and settled on our tattered couch in the living room with my confessors, the knife and champagne, to watch Frank Capra's masterpiece, *It's a Wonderful Life.* I'd rented my favorite film on the heels of my rejection from the Studio. It's a Christmas story with the syrupy message that each of us is an important soul and that we affect each other in ways we may never realize—Hollywood bullshit that some part of me longed to believe. If we are all the ages of ourselves layered 'round the littlest part of ourselves, like the rings that mark a tree's trunk, then the sapling in me adored the movie. I was a sap and knew it.

In a moment of dark despair, George contemplates suicide, which is waylaid by a dotty angel who shows him what the world would be like if he'd never been born. My mother raised me to believe in guardian angels, but I had considered her story a trick to get us kids out of her hair and into bed. I pondered what the world would be like if I'd never been born and decided it probably would have saved some heartache. I searched my past for good deeds and came up empty handed. I was drowning in a sea of self-pity and ashamed of myself for it.

Jimmy Stewart was so convincing. I'd reached the desperate moment in the nightmare scene when George sits at the bad bar praying for relief. Next moment, he's socked in the jaw and figures that's what he gets for praying. Dang, Stewart was gifted. I'd been told that I was a good actor too, and couldn't a fine one bring relief from the trials of life? Couldn't she elucidate our shared humanity? Maybe I hadn't caused only sorrow. I remembered the communion I'd felt during my first role as Irene in high school and my heart sank all over again about The Actors Studio. Terry Hayden materialized, "When are you going to take responsibility for your talent?" I drank another cup of champagne.

By the time George's life had been saved, I'd all but finished the bottle. Now I was confused about my roommates' schedules and fearful that one of them would show up to find me sprawled on the couch, in one altered state or another. Plans to camouflage the somnambulism with revelry had been boomeranging right and left. Even though I'd kept quiet about the night of Looking for Mr. Goodbar, Sandy, the girl who held the lease to our apartment and the most responsible of us, had pushed me to see her therapist. I agreed to a session, but after the woman questioned me about blackouts, I never returned. I saw asking for help as a one-way ticket to the looney bin. I was about to make sure that never happened.

I buried the empty bottle in the far reaches of my closet from where it came. I settled into my room with the last sips of champagne in one hand and the steak knife in the other. I locked the door.

I undressed and reclined on my futon. I could almost feel my sharp accomplice through the pillow, the princess and the blade. If only it could cut through my crap. I was unaware at the time that the root of the word *sarcasm* is the Greek *sarkasmos*—to tear flesh, to bite one's own lip in rage.

It was a muggy night and I couldn't afford an air conditioner. I remembered how my deceased neighbor at Eighty-First Street had stunk. My current room had been divided from a larger one and had no window. When I had first moved in, I'd hoped the quiet would help me sleep, but there was no shutting out the noise inside my head. I wondered how Piano Boy fared and lit my votive rose candle in his honor. It was not, however, the only light in my sham of a holy grotto. By this time, I kept a small bedside lamp on, day or night, to scare away the critters, both real and imagined.

I began to cry. I was not a bad girl, only weary beyond reckoning.

Angel of God, my guardian dear, to whom His love entrusts me here, ever this night be at my side to light and guard, to rule and guide.

I'd ventured the prayer in hopes of relief but only felt filthier inside and out. See, that's what you get for praying—just like George Bailey said. No amount of compunction could keep me from my sins. The previous night's insanity flooded me. I examined the digs on my forearms. I'd both received and inflicted similar wounds when Danny and I fought as kids. We would kick and scratch. We'd bite each other to the point of bleeding and twist the tender skin on the inside of each other's arms. When we got hurt from roughhousing, my mother used to say, "See, God punished you."

Somnambulism felt like both the crime and the punishment. I was relieved to be miles from my family with no chance of them seeing the mess I'd become. Mom and I wrote. She'd always hated cooking and her letters included long litanies about dining out and what she and my father had ordered. She was finally well enough to enjoy their empty nest. My missives brimmed with cheery anecdotes, lies really, about how close I was to my big break. Sometimes my mother would inquire as to how I was sleeping, and I fabricated scenes of heavenly slumber. Often she'd include a five-dollar bill in case I needed to hop in a cab. My taxi ride of the previous night flushed my face hot with shame.

What would it do to my parents, this task at hand? I thought about Billy, about how far he'd come and how happy he was with Sue.

I felt the full pains of being a phony. For penance, I clutched my unkempt hair into big fistfuls, nearly tugging it from my head, and dug the heels of my hands into my shut-up eyes. I thought I should be more remorseful and wished tears would flow. I would have hit myself about the head if I'd thought it would help. Maybe it would. I slapped my cheek and suddenly out popped a memory from the previous evening seemingly unrelated to the hallucinated pterosaur.

In it, I was standing in a crowd outside of CBGB's down on Bowery. As if in slow motion, my arm pulled high above my head readying a blow. It came down hard to slap a young woman across her unsuspecting face. With all the nastiness that occurred that night, slapping that girl bothered me the most. I wondered who she was and what she had done to deserve my violence. Most probably nothing, although I would never know since the memory stopped when the sting of my hand met her cheek.

I felt sleepy, as if the shameful incident was too much to consider, so I roused myself with a cigarette and checked on the blade. I lay on the futon and finally cried. I smoked and cried and cried and smoked. Eventually the decision I contemplated weighted my weary eyelids. That night, there wasn't enough nicotine in the world to keep me awake.

I dreamt that I was in jail for murder. I believed I was innocent but everyone else was convinced otherwise. I had no recollection of the heinous act. Michael Hoffman came to visit me and we were allowed to talk privately on the empty basketball court behind the building that housed the prisoners. It was an ancient complex and creepy men peered down at us from between bars. The sky was nearly black from an approaching storm, but we didn't care; we were overjoyed to be together. I hugged him repeatedly to prove he was real. Surely he would see that I was innocent. When I told him so, he nodded his head, but I saw that he didn't believe me and hadn't all along. It was the saddest feeling ever, awake or asleep. Tears poured down my face. I suddenly realized I'd been holding loose-leaf papers in my hand covered in my poetry, and in that moment of awareness, the wind picked up and blew my poems away. I knew then that all was lost.

I opened my eyes to flames a foot high and leaping greedily. But were the flames really leaping or was my sleep terror leaping? Stupidly, I grabbed the coffee mug and threw what was left of the champagne at the fire. *Floosh*. Futon flambé. Heat rushed my face. Earlier in the week, I'd been soaking my feet after a long night of waitressing and, too tired to empty it, had left the bucket of water in my bedroom. *Swoosh*. It saved me. We'd no smoke alarms, or none that worked that night. I opened all the windows in the place, grateful that my room-mates weren't there.

It makes sense that I'd wanted to burn my bed.

On Saturday, I wandered Manhattan as if I were homeless. I was in shock, further shock, stockpiled shock. Parts of the city were a ghost town on the summer holiday weekend; parts overflowed with kids running through open fire hydrants to cool off amid squeals of laughter and bursts of firecrackers. I didn't know which scenes made me feel lonelier.

Late afternoon, Jimmy stopped me outside the newsstand on Broadway and One Hundredth Street. He was a neighborhood fixture who reminded me of Billy, if Billy were older and a city mouse. Jimmy was middle-aged but appeared ancient. He was always disheveled, dirty really, with sweaty skin, intensified by the July temperatures. He wore thick, black-framed eyeglasses held fast to his bowed head with a wide elastic band. Despite the coffee he continually sipped, he was mellow and leaned crookedly on a pair of taped-up crutches. His most outstanding handicap was his legs. They splayed out in opposite directions from the knees down. But I supposed he had other less visible ailments. I wondered if he was a Vietnam vet. He never told me his story, but whatever he'd weathered had left his body broken and his spirit, amazingly bright. He often recited passages from poetry as I passed. We small talked whenever I bought the paper at his hangout. Customarily, I didn't linger. His frankness and piercing glance unnerved me.

Jimmy was the neighborhood seer.

"What's making you blue, Little One?" He held out his crutch to prevent me from passing without a hello, which had been my intention on the day after the night of the fire.

Little One was Jimmy's nickname for me. I'd never given it much thought but in the moment it was a tall glass of water to my parched soul. I stopped and faced him. He fixed me with a penetrating look and spoke slowly, deliberately, "Hush, my dear, lie still and slumber! Holy angels guard thy bed! Heavenly blessings without number, gently falling on thy head."

I cried hard. He did not try to stop me. A round of firecrackers busted nearby and my distress shook out of me like a dog shakes from a racket. I couldn't keep any of it bottled up and dared to share about the fire and that I wished I were dead.

Jimmy asked the newsstand man for a paper towel and I wiped my face and blew my nose while he clucked and hushed me. He took my dirty hand in his dirty hand and I let him. It was the first time I'd allowed anyone to really connect with me since Theo. All the other hands I'd loved and lost along the way, both dead and alive, seemed to rush to surround me and Jimmy, to create a circle of safety in my dangerous world.

"Each time we're born into this world, life is new." He paused, searching for the right words. "Life is like a new pair of shoes. It takes time to break them in."

His words made no sense to me and all the sense in the world.

"Are you acquainted with the *White Album*?"

I couldn't reply because it had been one of Michael's favorites and because of the dream I'd had of him before the fire, or maybe it had been a warning. I nodded my head.

"Good." He smiled. "You're a sensitive one, so . . ." and he looked right through me, "you know Harrison's guitar will always weep."

I cried with renewed vigor.

"It's not about stopping the weeping. The tree of life is a weeping willow, honey."

My laugh surprised me and I snorted my tears. He smiled and encouraged me to give my nose a good long blow.

"Someday you're gonna find a way to weep and love yourself too, all of yourself."

I thought about Jimmy's broken body and imagined what he must go through, yet every day he found a way to hobble down to the corner and perform his role as street prophet. I sobbed again for Michael.

"A boy I loved, who died . . . he loved that song."

"There it is," he said, as if we'd finally gotten to the bottom of things.

"I don't know how I'm going to ever find rest. I don't see a way out of this . . ." I motioned at the world.

"You don't have to see a way. You're being taking care of. Watched over. That boy and a whole slew of other folks got your back."

I covered my face with both my hands to hide my desperate desire for his words to be true.

"No, no, no, no . . . there, there, Little One. Almitas, my mother called them . . . little souls."

"Almitas," I managed between sobs, "little souls."

"People who've loved ya and crossed over."

I thought about the German shepherd puppy on the night of Looking for Mr. Goodbar and how the dream of Michael had seemed to save me from the fire. I thought about my grandmothers, who'd come to see me on the night of Fur Elise.

"What should I do? How will I know what to do?" I hiccupped and he grinned again.

"Go home, Little One, and get some rest. It'll come to you."

He motioned me toward my building with his crutch. I hugged him.

"Thank you," I whispered. "You're an angel."

"Ha!" he laughed, slapping his wrecked leg. "That's a good one!"

I went home. Too tired to fight anymore, a kind of peace had descended. My futon had been scorched beyond repair. I stretched out on the couch and slept through the night.

On Sunday, as I dragged my futon out to the sidewalk, I remembered that I'd made a date to walk through Riverside Park with a woman who worked at Circle-in-the-Square Theatre. Mary Maguire was in her late twenties and about to enter law school. A real grown-up. We were only acquaintances and I was flattered and curious why she'd asked to hang out with me. I didn't know it had been set up by a number of friends who'd been worried for months, including my teachers, Terry and Jackie, and my roommate, Sandy.

We met by Seventy-Second Street and strolled through the park. The humid weather was a dirty blanket and I hadn't had a drink since the night of the fire. My arms went numb as we strolled. I later learned that the sensation was a detox symptom.

Mary asked me about my drinking and I hedged. She told me that her father had been a wonderful man who'd turned into a violent drunk then turned back into a wonderful man after getting sober. We sat on a bench facing the Hudson and it felt like a dream. She was urging me to get help, and as she spoke, a story I'd heard at P&G's the week before went through my head.

It had been told by an elderly woman, a frail stranger who'd sat at the bar speaking aloud to anyone who would listen, but the regulars, the boys' club, ignored her. She wasn't young or pretty. She was invisible to them. It was toward the end of my shift, the night of her story, and I stood, exhausted, at the far end of the bar, waiting for Al to fill my order. She spoke softly, almost inaudibly with the noise of last call taking place. I was captivated and leaned in.

She had grown up with a father who was a real souse. One night he'd gotten it into his head to send the baby of his big family, a boy of five, into a dark room to find something he needed. The dad was keen on sadistic games and wouldn't allow him to turn on the light. The delicate lady couldn't recall what her littlest brother had been ordered to fetch but their dad had to have it. She begged to be allowed to help, but he only towered over her with bared teeth and screamed for the boy to hurry up. Her brother panicked then, in the darkened room. He'd been searching, searching the floor on all fours to find who-knows-what in an effort to please the drunk. He stood up fast and ran, face first, into a doorknob. It was an old-fashioned glass one, the lady noted sadly—hard and unforgiving. The boy lost his eye on account of it.

I burst into tears on the bench at the Seventy-Ninth Street Boat Basin. There was an awful lot of crying that lost and found weekend. Was this what Jimmy had meant when he'd said it would come to me, what to do? Mary put her arm around my shoulder and we sat like that for a long, long time.

I thought about how long I'd been fetching for a fight and how, like the P&G patrons, I'd been afraid to go home. The surprised face of the woman I'd slapped on the night of the imagined pterosaur floated before me, as well as the assailant's knife. A guy I'd started dating, a drinking buddy from the bar, had recently said to me, "If you hit me one more time, I'm going to hit you back." I'd worn a long sleeve shirt in the heat to cover the cuts on my arms from where I'd dug away my skin a few nights before, but I couldn't hide those wounds from myself.

Then there'd been my shameful contemplation of the ultimate self-violence. I'd thrown away my roommate's razor along with the singed futon earlier that morning. I didn't want to be violent toward myself or anybody else. "I'm alive, I'm alive!" George Bailey had hollered when he'd come out of his nightmare with his kids heaped about his neck gleefully. I'd always said that I never wanted children because I'd just fuck them up. But secreted away, deep in my heart, I wanted kids someday. And I didn't want to hit them, ever.

I looked across the bench at Mary and remembered when Bedford Falls gathered to save George from ruin.

A veil had lifted. Grace. Mysterious that.

Within a few weeks, with the help of like-minded drunks, I put down the booze and removed blackouts from the equation.

PART III: RECOVERY

Ring the bells that still can ring, forget your perfect offering
There is a crack, a crack in everything, that's how the light gets in.

Anthem, by Leonard Cohen

FIRST THINGS FIRST

I t's a mystery why some people find relief from addiction and others don't. It seemed to me that suffering had softened my stoic heart. Weariness had left me vulnerable to my friends' intervention. Whenever my dad talked about surrender in relation to being sober, he used the military definition—"to join the winning side." I'd grown sick and tired of searching for relief from sleepwalking in the bottle. I'd grown sick and tired of sleepwalking through my days.

As a kid, the booze seemed to settle my nerves and help me sleep. But it actually made me pass out, which is physiologically far from a healthy, restorative sleep state. A dearth of rest left me incapable of emotional growth and well-being. To say that alcohol served me until it turned on me would be a lie. It sickened me from the start. Mine was not a story of conviviality gone sour. Pissing my pants and blacking out the first time I drank at the age of twelve was not social drinking. In that blackout, I could have wandered into traffic crossing Route 9 the very first time I drank.

It took time to believe I deserved sobriety, that it wasn't a dream, too good to be true. I lacked faith and borrowed my friends'. They ascribed to Jimmy's philosophy that each of us was being cared for by a higher power of our own understanding. During those early days of abstention, while I shook and cried and detoxed, I resigned from the debate team over the God question. I leaned into the great mystery of life and kept my eyes open in earnest for any signs that brought me comfort and kept me away from the first drink.

I realized I'd always been searching for interconnectedness, even as a girl with my rosaries and scapulars.

July 29 is my sobriety date and my Grandpa Frazier's birthday. He was an alcoholic who died when my father was eleven. Dad shared only a few memories of him. One was during Prohibition. Dad was little—maybe seven or eight, and he would run through the alleys of Albany in the dark, a jar of hooch hidden in his jacket for Grandpa because he needed it. He had to have it. He couldn't sleep without it.

I took my sobriety date as a sign that Grandpa Frazier had my back. Almitas. I learned to keep the focus on myself and to save the one life I had some power to save. Eventually, I cleared up enough to realize that even though most alcoholics would not recover, we each deserve it. And I didn't deserve it any less than the next guy.

The end of blackouts was a huge relief. When I woke during sleep-walking, remembered flashes the next day, or was told by my room-mates that I'd walked, at least I knew that it was not from drinking. Insomnia is a symptom of alcohol withdrawal, but I had lived with it all my life.

What was new for me was the comradery during those long nights. My friends and I would hang out at twenty-four-hour diners and laugh over our narrow escapes. It was never gallows humor but rather the hilarity of sheer relief. And we cried. Big buckets of tears. We called ourselves the Upper West Side Water Brigade. I was still terrified that once my waterworks started they'd never stop, but my new friends assured me otherwise. I had to cry, they said, if I wanted to truly heal, to grieve the losses I'd stuffed with alcohol. One defi-nition of *comrade* is "a fellow soldier." We were winning our battles over addiction. We were stepping, however tentatively, out of dark isolation and into the light of our joining together. We were saving one another's lives.

When I was afraid to go to my rented room, afraid to go to sleep, especially if I'd recently had an episode, I'd stay at my sober friend's house. Beth, her husband, and their two daughters, who were nine and six at the time, showed me only kindness. I'd sleep in their living room on the pullout sofa. Being included, spending time, especially nighttime, with their family was amazing. They piloted me through many a dark night. We'd watch bad TV, eat popcorn, and play board games. Sometimes we would get into rousing rifts over charades or Trivial Pursuit. It felt safe to act like an adolescent stuck in a grown woman's body, which is what I was. They taught me about true intimacy—about being messy, being human, and being loved anyway. I never had a night terror at their house.

After my failed audition for The Actors Studio in 1985, my pack encouraged me to start the process all over again. By 1986, I'd been awarded a final audition and fashioned a piece from Steinbeck's *Wayward Bus*. My scene partner was Studio member Chad Burton. He played a bus driver who had intentionally careened into a rut on a desolate dirt road. I played a passenger, a college girl who was unhappy and searching for the meaning of life.

During a pivotal moment we sat on a bench, looking at the sunset, which meant facing the judges. The old desire to disappear descended but Chad is an actor's actor. Seeing my fear, he simply took my chin in his hand and turned my face to the fourth wall, to admire the sky. His generosity was contagious and my heart opened wide. A deep well of gratitude flooded my eyes. I connected with the audience and felt a greater power moving between us, like during my early days of theatre. I had dropped my armor on stage.

Every judge but two voted me in. Elia Kazan and Ellen Burstyn, whose decisions counted the most, did not. Maybe they remembered my awful audition the previous year. It's very tough to become a member of The Actors Studio—Harvey Keitel auditioned seven times—but based on that Steinbeck scene, I was invited to work in session throughout the following season. I did and was noticed. However, when the appointed time for the 1987 finals came around, I was a wreck.

My mom's cancer, which had been in remission for some years, had metastasized to her bones. By Memorial Day, she was admitted to hospice care at the Albany VA. My neck had gone out due to the stress. I felt and looked idiotic, sentenced by my doctor to wear a giant foam neck brace.

Exhausted and ashamed, I approached Ms. Burstyn after session— the week before finals. Would she think I was exaggerating my mother's illness because I was afraid of yet another failed audition? My voice shook but I managed to hold back the tears. I told her my mom was in hospice and asked if I could remain a finalist for another year and take my audition in 1988. "Of course," she said, "yes."

It broke my heart and my pride to ask for that extension. It was weakness to an independent girl. I couldn't see the strength in it; I didn't recognize the health. Asking for help was still a soft muscle. My love of acting, my love for the Studio, had afforded me the opportunity to lay down my armor on the stage, and I'd claimed the success. But this felt like failure.

I'd left P&G's when I'd stopped drinking and had taken a nine-to-five job as a switchboard operator at a travel agency. It gave me weekends free to visit my mom upstate. I stayed over at the hospice and slept on a cot beside her. I often startled awake from fear during my vigils, but as far as I know, I never had a severe sleepwalking or sleep terror episode. I sometimes cried, come morning, from the sheer relief of having not disturbed her during her final nights of rest.

The Saturday after asking to postpone my audition, I took the train to see my mother. I waited until evening, when we were alone, to tell her about the Studio. Mom had always championed my acting and I hated the idea of disappointing her. She followed the careers of many Studio members and understood how important it was to me and also the prestige of being selected. By this point, her bones were too brittle to leave her bed. I climbed in beside her.

"You're going to be a famous actress!" was her only reply.

Blubbering me, "It's not that . . ."

"What, you just want to work? You will—you'll work as an actress!"

Whimpering me, "It's not that . . ."

"What is it then?" Mom's eyes brimmed with tears, too.

Hiccuping, "I just want to grow along spiritual lines."

We burst out laughing in that contagious way when the reality of death trumps all.

When I returned to the city, I received a call from my friend, Mark Ethan. He's a member of the Studio who had worked on a scene with me in session. He'd snuck into the final auditions and reported to me that Ellen Burstyn had announced to the other judges that she would invite me to become a member based on my work with members in session. There were six of us selected that year, including Michael O'Keefe and Delroy Lindo. Because I was the only woman, we called ourselves the Mod Squad, as in the hippie, cop television show of the late sixties-early seventies.

I was so excited to share the happy news with Mom the following weekend. We poured over a newly published book, *The Actor's Studio: A Player's Place* by David Garfield, and giggled like schoolgirls. We were just getting to know each other as women. My sobriety had gifted us that, but cancer was about to snatch it away. I cried and my mother assured me she'd be okay, that she'd dreamt of being alone in a rowboat without oars, flowing on the gentle current of a river. A radiant lady floated in the air before her, showing her the way toward the brightest, most beautiful light she'd ever seen.

"I'm not worried about you, I'm worried about myself," selfish me. "Come here."

It was the middle of the night, a week before her passing. There was no climbing in beside her anymore, her bones were that fragile. I held her hand and kissed it. "You weren't making up guardian angels, were you, just to get us to go to sleep?"

She shook her head, no. "I'll be right with you, I'll be watching over you."

I told her about almitas and she smiled.

"I'll send you signs. I believe in them." Mom reminded me that the day of the bad news about Billy had been St. Dymphna's Feast Day and how it had helped her accept his mental illness.

"Maybe it was a sign from one of your almitas. Maybe it was a sign from your mom . . . she sure suffered her share."

"I'm so happy you're sober. I knew something was wrong but I didn't know what. Now it's like you're back. You've got that sweetness back. Like when you were a girl."

Mom wept and I lowered the bed railing and, ever so gently, leaned to her, cheek-to-cheek. She caught her breath and calmed down. She whispered, "I'm so sorry you inherited my very bad nightmares."

"I'm sorry you had them too, Mommy . . . don't forget . . . St. Dymphna is the patron saint of sleepwalkers, too."

She took up crying again. I hushed her but she wouldn't have it.

"No, no, Kathy. Let me say this . . . I'm so sorry about the . . . when we were . . . when we were, so . . ." Searching, searching for the words she could allow her heart to say between sobs. ". . . we had no idea what we were doing." We stayed beside each other and it was my turn to soothe her with the lullaby she'd created a lifetime ago.

Once I had a baby, a baby, a baby,
Once I had a baby, an old tomato patch.
And Mommy is that baby, that baby, that baby,
Mommy is that baby, that old tomato patch.

They say our lives flash before our eyes in facing our own death, but my mother's flashed before me that night. I realized the depth of her intelligence—how she'd read three newspapers a day; I felt her pride at having been a WAV during World War II, and nostalgia for her beautiful voice. She'd boasted a solo, "Ave Maria," sung as a girl at the Cathedral of the Immaculate Conception in Albany. Like most women of her generation, she'd given up her dreams to marry and raise kids.

My mother's amends illuminated my journey backward through time and rang 'round my heart—the heart I'd thought I'd left behind, buried in the foundation of my childhood home on Glennon Road. I felt the pain of her childhood as I stroked her hair and hummed her song. She'd been a lost and sleepless waif of a girl. Her mother's mental illness, her father's alcoholism had stalked her throughout her whole life in the form of sleep terrors. I was her "late in life" baby and she'd been bereft of any ability to offer nighttime comfort by the time I was born.

Leaning over, cheek-to-cheek with my mother as she lay in that hospital bed, we were transported back in time to when a lonely winter light reached through the living room picture window of our tiny Cape Cod. But it could not frighten me, not with the golden light from the table lamp that encircled my mother as she sat in our La-Z-Boy reading her newspapers. I must have been seven and could have stood there forever before being noticed, so deep was her interest in world events. She was an escape artist of sorts as she dove through those papers into more thrilling happenings, far from humdrum suburbia.

My mother had been beautiful with blue eyes and creamy skin—a movie star basking in her spotlight, only playing the part of a house-wife. She wore a muumuu over a T-shirt. No long, silky legs and heels. White anklet socks ballooned over her Hush Puppies. The neighbor-hood kids taunted me that she was fat, but I loved her softness.

"Mom?" I'd dared to interrupt her reading.

"Yes, honey?" she responded, peering through her bifocals at the *Albany Times Union*, turned at an angle to catch the light.

"Can you hold me on your lap?"

"Sure, Kitten, let me put my papers down." Neatly she'd folded them, never losing her place. Then she'd taken off her glasses, pearly blue-framed, being certain to rest them in their case. Her curvaceous arms opened to hold me close to her heart. She never said I was too old to cuddle during the day. I was happy for her roundness and her peachy skin. It didn't matter to me that her hands were stained with news ink or that they smelled like Clorox bleach from perpetual laundry.

"Will you sing me that song you used to sing me when I was little?"

"Sure, honey," and I sunk into her lap and the comfort of our lullaby.

Back then, it had been impossible for my mother to give any comfort once nighttime fell. You cannot give what you do not have, and leaning beside her in bed at the hospice, as her final darkness descended, I'd finally grown up enough to understand why.

The night before my mother's death, I was once again alone with her. I refused sleep. I didn't want to leave her even for a minute. What if she was alone when her time came? She moaned in her sleep. She'd been administered the optimal dose of morphine.

"What can I do?" I begged the hospice nurse. "Isn't there anything I can do?"

She could have dismissed me, shook her head, and shrugged her shoulder. But instead she brought a bowl of water and a wash-cloth. I sat beside Catherine Rose Tallmadge Frazier and turned the cool cloth on her forehead. She'd birthed me into this world, and I was helping to birth her into the next. I understood that this amends to my mother was also an amends to Michael. For the first time in my life, I wasn't leaving someone before they could leave me.

My mother remained unconscious. Well into the next night, our family gathered around. The hospice nurses told us when her time grew near.

"The mottling has begun. Feel her feet."

They were freezing, blotching blue and purple, her hands too. Death had taken a rope hold to climb her limbs and steal her from us. The final sleep.

My parents had celebrated their fortieth wedding anniversary on June 21. In the early hours of July 6, in the middle of the night, my father lay in a recliner asleep beside Mom's bed. As she took her final, rattled breaths, he talked in his sleep, begging repeatedly, "Where you goin', Kate? Where you goin'? Where you goin', Kate? Where you goin'?"

After my mother's death, back in the city, my friends rallied. The Actors Studio became a sanctuary. Terry Hayden and Jackie Brooks took special care of me. I participated in several workshops with one of the original members, Vivian Nathan. She said I was the salt of the earth and reminded her of Eva Gardner when she was young. Elia Kazan spent an afternoon interviewing me for the lead in a movie he'd hoped to direct—a sequel to *America, America*. He cast me but couldn't raise the money to produce the film. Ellen Burstyn became my mentor. She loves the Studio and has always nurtured young talent, but I was unprepared for her personal attention. In addition to encouraging me professionally, she mothered me in the face of my loss.

During my days, I made every effort toward improving myself as an actress. I left the switchboard job with the travel agency and waited tables again, to have more flexibility with auditions and jobs. My love affair with the theatre became all about the work. The stage is a place between two worlds, between art and life, between the players and the audience. I had traversed the worlds of asleep and awake for almost twenty years. My unconscious fascinated me. The intersections between my somnambulism and my acting fascinated me. I no longer feared my sensitivity in relation to a role. I began to understand how my emotions worked in that arena. But in real life, I could not corral my grief.

I wasn't afraid of the heartache over losing my mom but there was just so much of it. Every time I shared with my friends, I wept. One of them told me about CancerCare, a nonprofit that provides counseling to cancer patients and their families. I attended bereavement groups. But as I inched toward the first anniversary of my mother's death, sleepwalking and sleep terrors grew—once again, ferocious.

THE OPEN WINDOW

My long nightgown twisted around my ankles. I'd always hated that trapped feeling. I turned from side to side on the moldy couch in a ridiculous effort to get comfortable. The springs of the sofa were nocturnal animals. They poised patiently, waiting for the exact instant when my body surrendered to sleep so they could pounce up and bite me. I spent this particular night in the enormous living room of Bob and Jane's apartment to avoid the smell of paint drying in my rented postage stamp of a bedroom. Deep blue had been my color choice, having read it could calm the nerves.

Sandy and my other apartment mates had all left the city. Still resigned to communal living, I became one of several boarders in a rambling flat on the Upper West Side of Manhattan. My landlords were middle-aged Bohemians, writers, filmmakers. He was a philanderer. I'd played a Wild West saloon whore in a music video they'd made for a jazz saxophonist, which is how we became roommates. Their labyrinth halls led to disheveled rooms, some of which overlooked the Hudson with breathtaking views through windows left wide open in the unbearable summer heat.

I'd grown excruciatingly shy and barely knew the names of the other tenants who wandered the hallways en route from their bedrooms to one of the many bathrooms. Some of them hardly left their quarters. Others came and went quickly, keeping odd hours, reminiscent of my sublet with Theo. My room was in the back, off the kitchen, with a small, dirty window that faced an airshaft. Once the maid's room, it included a closet-sized bathroom with toilet and sink. I hated having to shower or bathe in one of the larger bathrooms, shared with strangers.

If sharing a bathroom unnerved me, the idea of bunking down in an open, common space, through which one or more of them would pass during the course of the evening, horrified me. I especially cringed at the idea of Bob creeping past me in the middle of the night upon his return from a liaison.

Despite condemning myself as juvenile, I'd plugged in my angel night-light nearby. I wore my best nightgown, too—lightweight and sleeveless but modest. Even in the dark, appearances mattered to me. It was the prettiest shade of rose pink, my mother's favorite flower and I wore it in Catherine Rose's honor. It was August 6, 1988, and would have been her sixty-eighth birthday. A month earlier had been a year since she died. I'd been attending a bereavement group at CancerCare the whole time, and it seemed to me that my grief should have eased after the one-year anniversary of my mom's death. Instead it weighed heavier than ever.

Green glow-in-the-dark numbers on my radio alarm clock flipped in slow motion.

I turned on a reading lamp and the sudden light sent a cockroach scampering across the hardwood floor beneath a huge, discarded pile of newspapers. How would I ever fall asleep with the fear of the disgusting creatures crawling all over me at my most vulnerable?

I banished the thought by picking up C. S. Lewis's *The Screwtape Letters* about a senior demon's correspondence to his nephew on how to damn a man. I read until my eyes felt heavy. I let them close, resting the Devil's letters against the *thump, thump, thump* of my heart. Blood pulsed through my ears. As a kid, I'd listened to that dreadful sound for what seemed like hours as I tried to fall asleep.

I realized, as I was about to drift off on the lumpy sofa, that these were not the most soothing bedtime thoughts. Reaching to turn out the light, I changed my mind and left it on. I must have fallen asleep then. I don't know for how long.

I came to in the middle of it, like waking inside a horror movie, silent scream and all. Eyes wide open. I was standing at an open window, staring at the dizzying curve of Riverside Drive, five floors below. I'd stopped, somehow, poised, about to jump. My beating heart told me so. Sweat streamed down the sides of my face and between my breasts. I had grasped the window frame with both hands. My adrenaline was so high, I could have lifted it off the wall. It was a big window, a portal from this world to the next. A solitary street lamp cast a pool of yellow light on the winding street. No cars. The air was thick.

I was alone. Or was I?

My mind raced, searching, searching for the truth. I'd been fleeing something real.

Oh my God, it had bitten me.

I backed a step away from the window and swiped furiously at my bare arm, as if I could swipe my terror away. That was it. Disgusting. Dirty. A rat had bitten me, sinking its sharp teeth into my upper arm. It had been real. I remembered seeing it clearly, filthy and gray. I remembered the weight of it, tricking me awake with its tickling whiskers.

I felt my arm for blood but there was none. I stared long and hard but my skin was smooth, unmarked. If only I could relax and think, master what was real. My nightgown, soaked in perspiration, clung to my skin. It was an all too familiar feeling. *Stupid, stupid girl.* I grabbed my hair and pulled it hard. I clutched my head and begged my mind to figure, figure out what had transpired. All of this happened in a flash, but not for me. I could not find my way back, search as I may.

I must have run from the couch across the huge expanse of living room to escape some nightmarish rat that had bitten through my sleep. I could not catch my breath, standing there at that open window, no screen, black night waiting, always waiting.

And then it dawned on me, and as surely as I had been convinced there had been a rat, minutes later I knew there had never been one at all.

Everything unraveled faster then. My hands still stung from where they'd slapped the frame. The window was tall as a door and wide as an invitation, but this frame had stopped me from leaping the five stories.

Then the shaking began, like a dog shakes terror from her body.

I cowered my way across the enormous room. I couldn't take my eyes off the window and backed up all the way to the tattered sofa in the corner where, moments before, I'd been fast asleep. I sat on the edge of that raft of a couch and clung to my pillow for dear life. I trembled and cried for what felt like a long, long time. The apartment was still. The city street was quiet. It felt like I was the only person awake in the whole world.

A breeze blew across the room and shivers climbed my spine despite the heat. I stared at the void beyond the open window. I squeezed my pillow even tighter as the reality of the situation hit me, really hit me—if I had fallen to my death while sound asleep, it would have been considered suicide. Was there some part of me that had dreamt the rat attack as an excuse to leap? It was too awful to consider. I was a cat trapped in a sack, drowning in my self-made river of fear. Any mention of it to anyone, ever, would lead to involuntary commitment.

I hadn't the slightest idea how to transport myself from the precipice I faced that night to safe ground. But there was one thing I did know: I was an Irish American girl, raised to white-knuckle unsavory problems alone. My heart beat fast again, caught in a body with a mind of its own.

"I was only sleepwalking . . . it was just a night terror," I whispered to no one there.

What I really wanted was a good, stiff drink. If this had happened in a movie, surely the heroine would be offered a shot to calm her nerves. But I was not an ingénue in a film. Even half-awake, I knew that my real life efforts to self-medicate the sleep disorders with liquor had failed miserably. I hadn't touched a drop in three years and had quit cigarettes for almost as long.

I wrestled with my shame on the ratty couch. As I stayed sober, shouldn't I be sleeping better and better instead of worse and worse? This whole thing was obviously my fault. I was too emotionally sensitive or repressed, or resentful. I was spiritually bereft, self-centered. I was immature and wouldn't accept my mother's death. I couldn't let go. I'd mentioned to my bereavement counselor about the return of my night terrors. "It's not uncommon during grief to experience night terrors or nightmares," he said, lumping the words together, "Have you tried yoga?" I had—I'd been practicing since college.

The medical community remained in the dark, same as me. I was defenseless against the episodes. *Tolerate* was still the only option I knew. The exhausting reality of my illness colored everything, every relationship in my life. My most recent boyfriend had broken up with me. He never said it was because of my sleepwalking, but one night, as I screamed him awake, he screamed back at me, his face twisted with torture, "I can't take this anymore!"

I had to find some way to rest, which seemed ludicrous after this night's episode. I had an early workday ahead of me, a Sunday brunch shift at J. G. Melon's. The weekend before, that same shift had been frantically busy and I'd been so exhausted that, while winding my way through the crowded tables of the back room, I spilled a tray of Bloody Marys and mimosas all over a customer's power-suit jacket. The lady called me an idiot, and although my cheeks burned hot, I felt it was an accurate description of my mental condition. Luckily, the manager was forgiving and my only consequence was a stern warning and to pay for the woman's dry cleaning. Later, as we counted our tips, my fellow waitstaff and I dubbed the slip, Sunday

Bloody Sunday, as in the U2 song. Despite my false bravado and the other waiters' efforts to make light of the incident I couldn't afford to mess up again or I'd surely be fired.

I reconsidered the nightcap.

No.

I prayed, *God grant me the serenity to accept the things I cannot change, the courage to change the things I can, and the wisdom to know the difference.*

Then the strangest thing happened—a thought I'd never had before when waking up, all alone in the middle of an impossible episode, popped into my weary head. Even though it was four o'clock in the morning and I was a freak, maybe, just maybe, I could call someone. We sober drunks were always calling each other. I would never dare tell all. Still, maybe I could call. Ridiculous. Who would be awake and who could I trust? I thought of my insomniac neighbor and gentlest man in the world. The Birdman.

Henry was in his late fifties and retired on disability. He'd been a night-shift worker who suffered from adult-onset Myotonic Muscular Dystrophy. One symptom was excessive sleepiness during the day with insomnia at night. He was up from pain too. My friend kept dozens of delicate birds in his single-room occupancy for company. MMD had rendered him excruciatingly slender, and when he walked, his knee joints hyperextended, causing a strange birdlike gait. With each step, he flapped his arms, bent at the elbows, to prevent a fall. Even his features were aquiline and his skin yellow, like one of his beloved finches or parakeets.

Bob and Jane had an ancient, black rotary phone that sat on the end table beside the couch. That night, it was the heaviest phone in the world.

When Henry answered, I attempted, between sobs, to tell him most of what had happened. I did not reveal the truth about the window. I was petrified that he would call 911 and the men in the little white coats would cart me away to Bellevue. I shook from making the call. Fear of being committed consumed me—of course it did. But Henry knew his own kind of darkness and he knew that I was in real trouble.

He listened. Although I could hardly make out his cooing words through my tears, I was comforted by the cadence of his voice and by the birds chirping through the silences. He knew to stay on the phone with me for as long as it took to talk me down. I finally heard the words he'd kept repeating.

"You don't have to be alone with this anymore."

I wanted to believe him, and my friend meant well, but I knew better. I promised Henry that I would return to sleep even as I knew it for a lie. Just like I'd left out the part about ending up at the open window, poised to jump.

Eventually I had to hang up the phone and manage the rest of the night on my own, mind racing. I'd been waking up more frequently during the onslaught of episodes since I'd lost my mom. Usually, afterward, sleep would descend like in the poppy scene in *The Wizard of Oz* when Dorothy and her friends are drugged into slumber by the Wicked Witch, only I refused to surrender to the spell during the night of the open window. I don't know how long I sat up before my eyes shut against my will and I immediately felt the threat of the imagined rat or some other terror, patiently waiting to pounce.

One more year until the relief of thirty—still, schizophrenia seemed as close as the open window. I stood and dared to walk to it. I intended to shut it, to lock out the night. Instead I looked out onto the world. The sky eventually brightened and the city yawned awake. Henry's assurance of not having to be alone with this anymore turned out to be correct: my oldest, most dependable companion had returned—a feeling of impending doom. It engulfed me. As sure as the day dawned for the rest of the town, I knew what waited for me at the end of that tired day and the next, and the next.

PLEASE, SIR, MORE?

Henry insisted on taking me out to dinner that Sunday night to one of our favorite hole-in-the-wall diners, Happy Burger on Broadway. A drawing of Mr. and Mrs. Happy Burger, people with smiling burger heads, decorated the menu. He steered me toward the back booth. I felt ten years old and worried about a scolding. I couldn't eat so I sipped tea. We sat facing each other and it was hard to hold my friend's gaze. Maybe it had been a mistake to share my shameful rat terror. But Henry was smart. He did all the talking.

He told me all about his newest blue parakeet named Sky and how she was the sweetest puff of cloud he'd ever seen. I loved hearing him share about the delicate birds and the comfort they gave him. He was in pain all the time from the MMD. He had emphysema, too, from years of smoking; although, he'd quit by the time I met him. Like me, he once set his bed on fire while drinking and smoking but hadn't been so lucky. His right arm and that side of his jaw and neck were scarred with thick, leathery, grafted skin. After the Birdman finished gushing over Sky, he made me snort my tea with a story about his parrot, Pickles, who picked up colorful phrases from MTV. By the time he finished his spanakopita, I felt much better. Better enough to order a piece of cheesecake.

I'd gotten through my brunch shift at J. G. Melons without any spills, but now my hands shook when I held my cup out for the waitress to pour more hot water. The little orphan boy, Oliver, came to mind—the moment when he dares to present his bowl for more gruel. I was an orphan girl stuck inside a woman's body since my mother's death. I didn't want to bother anybody. I didn't want to ask for more. Henry's attention on the phone the previous night had been enough. I didn't think I could stand another cup of kindness.

"What are we going to do with you?" he asked as we waited for the dessert.

"Let them eat cake," I barbed, dunking my tea bag.

"Wasn't so funny last night."

"They always seem worse in the moment." I waved my spoon nonchalantly.

"I hate the fucking night terrors."

"You get them?" If he'd told me the night before, I hadn't heard him.

He nodded and looked away. My cheesecake had arrived and he didn't want the waitress to hear. The kitchen bell rang and she turned to leave us, but not before topping Henry's coffee and giving him a wink. All the ladies found him irresistible.

"I didn't know that, Henry. I'm sorry."

"My dad was a violent man, a drunk. Night terrors are pretty common, you know, in alcoholic homes."

He knew my story . . . somewhat . . . but what had I said about my family in the wee, small hours of the night? *Don't ever share what goes on inside this house*, my mom's voice echoed from the far reaches of my childhood.

"God, that's terrible. I'm so sorry, Henry . . ." And then a spoonful of sugar later, ". . . my father hasn't touched alcohol for thirty years so I never saw him drink." Of course my friend sensed my defensiveness.

"It's nobody's fault . . . not if you believe it's a sickness."

171

"I get it, the hereditary thing, Henry, both my parents came from it, but what does hitting your kids have to do with your genes?" I imagined a little Henry cowering from a blow and it infuriated me. I pushed the cake away a little too hard.

"It's a family disease, emotional, physical, and spiritual. My father was just repeating what he'd learned. He'd been slapped around, too."

All of a sudden I'd left the conversation. His words had hit me upside my head and dislodged ancient slaps, historical slaps, inter-generational slaps. Sometimes my family had hit openhandedly, sometimes with a fist. We kids even played a game called Slap. The slapee would hold his hands out flat and the slapper would hold his palms up underneath but not touching. The slapper then tried to slap the slapee before he could pull away. It wasn't a contest of reflexes, like Hot Hands. We meant to hurt each other.

Once, Danny had slapped my hands raw-red. I was transfixed and couldn't simply walk away. I deserved it. I was weak if I couldn't stand it. It was love to us. Eventually, I busted out crying for help, Mom lumbered in, and the chase was on. She caught up with him on the stairs to the second floor and dragged him down by one foot with me begging mercy for my brother and Mom asking if I was happy now.

I remembered my father slapping me because I'd said *goddamn it* at the age of twelve. He threatened with his fist, *I ought to skin you alive*, and I wet my pants. Then how Mom spanked me when I was tiny, with the metal spatula for I don't know why. The nights I took refuge in my sisters' room when my parents fought, the sounds of yells and objects breaking reverberating up the radiator where I sat, hypnotized by the row.

Worst of all was when I was nineteen, the time when Danny was hung over and had called me a bitch. Something had come over me and if I could have slapped it out of him—the violence that stalked our family—I would have. Mom used to quote the Bible, "He who lives by the sword, dies by the sword." I had always felt that I deserved that black eye. It was terribly, terribly shameful and

I'd pushed it from my memory for so many years. It came flooding back, vividly triggered by Henry's words, I almost felt the throb of my swollen face.

My mind froze from the avalanche of remembered blows. Suddenly I was crying in that back booth of Happy Burger with the Birdman sitting beside me, his arm around my shaking shoulder. He'd seen me disappearing before his very eyes and had changed seats to be near me, to call me back. Invisible Woman was busted.

"Let us love you until you learn to love yourself," Henry whispered my favorite saying.

"It was true, what I said about my dad."

"I know . . . I know, Kathleen," he cooed.

"We were the only kids in the neighborhood who ran to meet their father when he came home from work. He worked so hard for us. The skin on his knuckles would crack from the cold . . . from delivering beer in all kinds of weather . . . delivering *beer*, Henry."

He cocked his head and tsk-tsk. "That's a lot for one of us."

"He'd get down on one knee when he stepped into the kitchen . . . arms wide open . . . Danny and I would run straight into his embrace."

"That's a lot of love."

"Both of them, Henry, both of them came from it . . . from the drinking. The rage would come over them, like a fit . . . like you said, Henry . . . like a sickness."

My friend held me and I cried for a long time. He told me that alcoholism is a chain forged link by link, generation by generation, gaining strength over time. He said that I was right . . . that my dad was the bravest man in the world and my mom, too . . . to have broken the chain that had threatened to strangle our family.

"You're lucky . . . blessed."

When I'd calmed down sufficiently, Henry walked me home. As we strolled slowly up West End Avenue, he told me about a program at St. Luke's-Roosevelt Hospital's Outpatient Addictions Center. It offered group therapy for adult children of alcoholics.

"Just think about it," he said as he hugged me goodnight. "And don't hesitate to call me if you need to . . . anytime, okay?" I nodded yes.

He'd planted the seed in perfect timing. My release had softened me enough to listen, if not commit.

I was relieved to find the stink of drying paint had dissipated in my back room at Bob and Jane's. I could never again sleep in that living room. My fear of roaches in proximity to their filthy kitchen waned in comparison to that open window. If this had once been the maid's room, it didn't give her much light, just a slit facing the backs of other buildings. I closed and locked it anyway, fell onto my futon, and fell asleep quickly. I slept soundly that night; my conversations with Jimmy and Mary seemed a lifetime ago. Kindnesses. Respites for my weary soul. They'd opened windows in my mind to let in light and air. Group therapy for adult children of alcoholics. Maybe my friend was onto something.

On Monday morning, I woke up feeling okay for the first time in a long time until I remembered what had happened Saturday night. I was off from work and dreaded the empty day before me. I decided to stay in bed. Even with the sun fully up, it was dusk-dim in my room. Any flutter of hope from the previous night had flown home with the Birdman. The idea of sitting in a circle, led by a therapist, and telling the truth terrified me. A stepping-stone to being committed.

I was thirsty and sipped water, wishing for something stronger. Henry's words returned, *it's nobody's fault . . . not if you believe it's a sickness*. I pulled the sheet over my head despite the heat and lay there for a long time, wishing I was dead. My ancestral alcoholism weighed heavy on my chest, a boulder to a condemned witch, and threatened to press the life out of me. I thought about the countless women who'd been accused of witchcraft over the years. It mattered little if they'd been guilty or not. If they refused confession, they would have been pressed to death. If they confessed, they would have hanged. Again it seemed to come down to quickly or slowly, how each of us would die. I wished for sleep. I wished for death. I whispered to no-one-there—

To die-to sleep-
No more; and by a sleep to say we end
The heartache, and the thousand natural shocks
That flesh is heir to. 'Tis a consummation
Devoutly to be wished. To die-to sleep.
To sleep-perchance to dream: ay, there's the rub!
For in that sleep of death what dreams may come
When we have shuffled off this mortal coil,
Must give us pause. There's the respect
That makes calamity of so long life.

Lying under my sheet on the Monday morning after the night of the open window, I considered a conversation my father and I had on the day my mother died. Standing alone together at the bedrail of her hospital bed, he'd whispered about how in 1928, when he was ten, his dad suffered a tragic car accident, and the surgeon put a steel plate in his head to hold his skull together. After that, he read the newspaper upside down. As his condition worsened, he didn't recognize my father or his older brother. Dad spent many nights lying awake from the sounds of his father's moans and his mother's sobs.

A year passed and Grandpa's health deteriorated further. Grandma sent my father (she called him Billy) away for a break with close family friends in Long Island. When his father died, his caregivers followed my grandmother's instructions and hid it from him, in an effort to protect him. They told him that his dad was doing poorly and took him home straight away. As he rode the train up to Albany, he was sad that his father was sick, but happy that he'd see him again soon. He played with toy soldiers on the seat of the train. Before the accident, Grandpa had called my father his little warrior on account of his love for those figurines. He wanted to be a brave boy.

When the cab pulled up in front of his apartment building, black crepe hung on the door and his heart sank. He knew it meant someone had died. He guessed it was his father, but didn't want to believe it. They lived in the top flat and, stair after stair, he climbed, two at a time, gaining momentum with each step, opening each family's door to see if it was their loss. When he got to the top and flung the door wide, there was his father's body laid out in mourning on the table.

"I don't think I ever got over that blow," he said back when we'd stood vigil by my mother's deathbed. I put my arm around him then, thinking about how that little boy was still inside my six-foot-three father.

Then he confided that his worst fear was of falling down a flight of stairs and breaking his neck. He listed a few people he'd known who had met that demise. One was a relative who'd been drinking at the Kiwanis Club. Then Dad realized that everyone he knew who died that way had been drunk. We hugged, relieved that our chances of a violent stair death were lessened considerably by being sober. In the moment, neither of us had remembered my near-fall down the stairs while sleepwalking as a teenager.

And now there was the incident of the open window.

With the sheet still over my head like a dead girl, my heart pounded as though I was standing at the window still. I was overwhelmed by my own close call and couldn't sift my story from my family's saga. I longed to believe in free will. It had seemed a real possibility as I'd sat at Happy Burger with Henry's arm around my shoulder. But alone in this old, maid's room, I believed in fate and feared it. It was only a matter of time before I slipped, driven to drink by the terrors. Or would they take me first? Should I confess or not? I had no idea what I should be confessing to.

As a kid, I used to make up sins as I knelt in the dark box, staring through the grate at the priest. I never owned up to any real transgressions, tattling on Danny, betraying him to Mom's rage, letting Billy take the blame when I scratched *fuck* into our basement door. I hadn't trusted the sanctity of confession. I figured, if I could recognize the priest (and I could), he probably recognized me too. The thought of the truth reaching my parents had been too terrifying to consider.

Around the time of the open window, some emotional memory work I'd been exploring at The Actors Studio had been bothering me—maybe the ferocity of my nocturnal wandering *was* a kind of internalized self-violence. Henry's counsel seemed to confirm it.

I was a ticking time bomb set to explode at my most vulnerable, as I lay sleeping. This tape will self-destruct in five seconds. *Mission Impossible*. How could I defuse my explosive self, all alone and in the dark as I was? It seemed futile to follow my friend's lead even as I picked up the phone and called St. Luke's-Roosevelt.

GET UP, IT'S TIME TO WAKE UP

After the night of the open window, I left Bob and Jane's to move into a much better situation. Nancy was a fellow actor, writer, and friend who owned the second-floor apartment on Ninety-Eighth and Broadway with a mile-long hallway, rooms to the left. I'd been room hopping in Manhattan for almost ten years and, as usual, mine was claustrophobic but not only because of its tiny size. Its singular window faced an alley directly above the exhaust fan of Ray's Pizza Parlor. I kept it closed, mostly because of the smell, but also because of the roar of their industrial-sized fan.

Many classmates from Circle-in-the-Square became working actors and some met real success. I acted in project after project at The Actors Studio. I scoured *Backstage* and attended open calls. I tried to see agents and to join any of the three acting unions, to no avail. I taught drama in a values education program in Long Island and continued waiting tables. I dated, at arm's length. I'd become, once again, a functioning somnambulist—mostly.

I'd turned down a tour with an educational theatre company. I said it was because I wanted to stay in the city, to be available for better acting work. But really, I was afraid to share a room. There would be no nightcap. Unfamiliar circumstances triggered episodes and I had to keep those to myself, as much as possible. Suppose I was housed on a high floor and wasn't as lucky as the night of the open window?

There were six of us in my group at St. Luke's-Roosevelt's outpatient clinic, and we met weekly with a therapist who was also an alcoholism counselor. Every single one of us had survived childhood violence and every single one of us suffered from insomnia, sleepwalking, night terrors, and/or narcolepsy.

The narcoleptic hid her illness from the group for a long time. She'd been particularly afraid of her employer finding out and of losing her job. She finally shared the severity of her situation between sobs. She had nodded off while driving over the George Washington Bridge. No accident had occurred but she was devastated. A sleep disorder center was recommended but she stopped attending group soon after her confession. I never knew what happened to her. As for the rest of us, I don't remember any referrals. I do remember one of our mantras— *nobody ever died from lack of sleep*—such was our ignorance and denial.

Childhood memories flooded. Everyone else's histories seemed far worse than mine. Their stories were black holes—mine, potholes. For a year and a half, I showed up faithfully. For a year and a half, somnambulism showed up faithfully. I shared selectively about sleep terrors, always minimizing their effects, especially if the episode had included walking. After all, we sat in a therapeutic room of St. Luke's-Roosevelt Hospital. The psych unit was painfully close. Despite my half-assed disclosures, I acted all bound and determined to get to the bottom of whatever caused the incidents. I would root it out. But the deeper I dug, the further I fell into my nightly hole.

Screams often woke my roommate, flashes of remembered incidents startled me from my days, or I'd awake in the middle of episodes. The latter happened more and more frequently. If I came to completely, I'd bumble to the kitchen with my flashlight afterward and eat cereal, often by the light of the cracked-open refrigerator. The bowl shook in my hands. Sometimes I spilt milk. Sometimes I cried over it. Eventually I would calm. The ritual grounded me.

It proved that I was alive and of this earth, not buried alive by my own unconscious hand.

Then I began having two episodes nightly, the first about an hour after falling asleep and the second at around four in the morning. Despite my guardian angel night-light, I would flee my bed to flick the light switch on the wall, always in an effort to escape whoever was coming to get me. I'd stopped leaving a reading lamp on because the light aggravated the insomnia and the insomnia aggravated the sleepwalking.

Nothing lifted my spirits like a candle in my rose candleholder. More than once, Nancy scolded me through my locked bedroom door as I was about to drift off to sleep or back to it— "Kathleen, you don't have a candle lit in there, do you?"

"No," I'd lie as I blew it out, fanning the smoke guiltily. I dreaded the possibility of another fire. Suppose I knocked it over during an episode? Suppose I wasn't so lucky this time, like Henry or worse? Suppose something happened to my roommate or neighbors? Still, I couldn't stop it.

I had continued to sleep on a futon, as a safety precaution, to be nearer the floor. In May 1990, at the age of thirty, and nearly five years sober, I fell to a show of false bravado and purchased a used bed from an actress who was moving to LA. The added height was an invitation for catastrophe. I snubbed my worry and pretended the purchase was a reward. I had, after all, survived my twenties without the diagnosis of schizophrenia. Henry used to say, "Act as if," and I loved the line from, *Field of Dreams*, "If you build it, they will come." Maybe if I started acting as if I were a normal sleeper, the sandman would come. There was no frame, just a queen-sized box spring and mattress that took up most of the room, wedged between two dressers.

I felt euphoric the first night as I lay down on my big-girl bed. My sheets were old, nearly threadbare, but just laundered and smelled of fabric softener. Mom had sent them to me from her linen closet when my marriage failed. I'd left all the wedding presents with Don and that suited me fine. These were much better anyway, old-fashioned with their cherry-colored stripes softened to a pastel pink from years of washing. Everything seemed to last longer back then. Or maybe I just couldn't let them go.

I was exhausted from a double shift at J. G. Melons and took it as a good sign that I fell asleep right away, until two pigeons startled me into panicked waking. They were fighting and fluttered frantically outside my window. A bad omen. Then I was up, despising the dark. It was one o'clock.

The bed would not fix me. Henry's health was in serious decline; I would not disturb him. Nancy slept soundly down the hall. I thought to call Beth and invite myself over but shame rose. They would certainly be sleeping, anyway. Besides, it would be an admission of defeat, and this was only my first night on the new/used bed. . . . Not that Beth or her family cared. It was me. I cared. I should have been beyond the ache, the longing of comfort from someone or something outside of myself.

My dream of a magic bed had turned out to be a hoax—and me, the con artist. I'd obviously retained nothing from my job as a magician's assistant. If only I could revive Invisible Girl and make myself disappear into the folds of my comforter nightly to reappear refreshed with the dawning of each new day.

I gave in and turned on a reading lamp. I'd been working on the Scottish play at the Studio with fellow member Brian Mallon—the scene when Lady Macbeth bullies her husband to screw his courage to the sticking post.

I got out my script and mask. I'd made the choice that my character had been flirting with the king and his men, warming to his guards before drugging them into thick stupors. The part whimsical, partly spooky half-mask that smacked of a she-goat in heat was the perfect prop. Nancy was amazing with a hot glue gun and had helped me make it from fur and wool and wooden horns.

I placed the mask over my face and looked in my full-length mirror. I wore a white nightgown. Chills ran the length of my spine. I'd loved mask work since college, when I'd studied with a woman who had studied with Decroux in France. He was the father of corporeal mime, which was not about showing the audience that you are stuck in a box. It was metaphor-based physical theatre, at its best a thing of real, sometimes unbearable beauty and power.

I left the mask on and read over all the lines that referred to sleep, or lack thereof, in the play. I'd highlighted them. They fascinated me, along with Lady Macbeth's sleepwalking. This was my favorite passage of Macbeth's:

Methought I heard a voice cry "Sleep no more!
Macbeth does murder sleep" —the innocent sleep,
Sleep that knits up the ravell'd sleave of care,
The death of each day's life, sore labour's bath,
Balm of hurt minds, great nature's second course,
Chief nourisher in life's feast.

Lady Macbeth tried nightly to rub the guilt from her hands. I ran from my imagined assailants, from their violence. Or was I running from my own? Her story ends in death—suicide we surmise—but we never find out how, and I decided it was while sleepwalking. I imagined her fleeing from a castle precipice, her nightgown billowing white as she fell.

She should have died hereafter;
There would have been a time for such a word.
Tomorrow, and tomorrow, and tomorrow
Creeps in this petty pace from day to day
To the last syllable of recorded time;
And all our yesterdays have lighted fools
The way to dusty death. Out, out, brief candle!
Life's but a walking shadow, a poor player

That struts and frets his hour upon the stage
And then is heard no more. It is a tale
Told by an idiot, full of sound and fury,
Signifying nothing.

A car honked a warning down on the avenue. I'd been reading for a long time. I put aside the play and removed my mask. My clock's digits glowed 4:00 a.m. How long until I realized that I could not outrun my fears while sound asleep? What would it take to make me stop my deadly dashes between the worlds?

I noticed that I hadn't fastened the latch on my bedroom door. I got up and locked it, for safety's sake—safety from myself, from my ramblings. Ridiculous, since a lock had never stopped me. I climbed back into my disappointment of a bed. It was hot for May—locked into that cramp of a room. But I hadn't slept with an open window since the night of the open window. I pushed off my stupid, old sheets. Defeated, I turned off the light. Was it trickier to see my denial in the dark?

My guardian angel night-light cast strange shadows on the goat mask sitting nearby. I was afraid of those shadows. I was afraid of my own shadow. Against all reason, I lit the candle in my rose candleholder.

Doctor: *How came she by that light?*
Gentlewoman: *Why, it stood by her. She has light by her*
     continually. 'Tis her command.

I'd been in a deep sleep when I was struck with the certainty that someone was coming to get me. The rest of what happened is unclear, stitched together from circumstantial evidence and remembered bits and pieces as they surfaced, very much after the fact—a film slipped loose from its reel.

I had to get to the light. A dog's legs jerk in response to her little doggie dreams but mine took me up and at 'em. I sprang from the bed I'd hoped would save me and ran for my life. But there was nowhere to go with those dressers, menacing sentinels hovering over me. I must have dashed full force, head first, into the one nearest the light switch. I was a bull, taunted by the red flag of my anger. The blow to the top of my head brought me to my knees. I collapsed fully, in slow motion. My jaw hit the floor first—a good right hook to my chin. Two-fisted floor, my nose was bashed next. Or was it the Irish American boxer in me? Our legacy. And our code of silence.

Kathy is so quiet, you wouldn't know she was here.

My phantom sparring partner—me, myself, and I.

I was down for the count.

Had I tasted the blood in my mouth?

The sensation of letting it go, of letting it all go completely, must have been inviting. For a moment I was stuck between two worlds, between the urge to pass out and a counter-pull toward consciousness. The candle flickered nearby. My mask witnessed the monumental struggle.

Somehow I woke up. I was kneeling and staring down at a puddle of blood. The floor swayed beneath me. When I looked up, I was startled by my mugged face staring back at me from the full-length mirror on my bedroom wall.

I didn't know what hit me, yet it was a blow for which I'd been braced. After all, I'd been fleeing my bed while sound asleep for twenty years.

I could have just as easily passed out and bled to death, alone and slumped on the floor of my tiny room. In those pivotal moments collapsed between the worlds of asleep and awake, I've often wondered if the littlest part of me, a life-loving girl, stirred inside of me. A quickening.

Get up, it seems she called, *get up. It's time to wake up.*

After I don't know how long, I unlocked myself from my room and stumbled the long, dark hallway to Nancy's. Her window faced east, toward Broadway. The day was just beginning to dawn. I stood at the edge of her bed. She was sleeping soundly. I hated to disturb her even as the blood pooled in my open hands. Could I convince her it was a nose bleed?

"Kathleen?"

"I had an accident . . . I had an accident."

"Oh, my God. Oh, my God . . . how? What happened?"

Only tears. No words from me.

The front of my nightgown was crimson. She quickly guided me to the bathroom, grabbed a towel, and held it under my chin. She ran cold water and directed me to rinse my hands. I rubbed them. *Out, damned spot! out, I say. . . . Yet who would have thought the old man to have had so much blood in him?* I would have laughed at the absurdity but for my fear of Nancy calling 911 and being dragged away to Bellevue.

She turned my face upward, toward the bright ceiling light, interrogation style. "What happened, what happened?" she repeated several times. She'd been shocked from sleep. I'd been shocked from sleep. Every inch of me trembled. I squinted up at the bare bulb. This was the stalking sin. How could I confess? I'd been tortured, beaten by my own hand—still I would not name names. I winced in pain when she gently dabbed a wet washcloth at my top lip where the bottom tooth had pierced. The bleeding ebbed. One top front tooth was so loose, I worried about spitting it out into my hand. I had recurring nightmares in which my teeth or shards of them fell from my mouth.

Finally I spat out, "I had an accident . . . sleepwalking," then stepped away from her. I had to step away from her.

"You have to go to the emergency room," I'm sure my roommate spoke kindly, but it meant punishment to me. The day had come. The day had finally arrived.

I howled, "I can't . . . I can't . . . I don't have health insurance," and it was true. But all I could see in my mind's eye was me, strapped into a straitjacket, same as Billy so many years ago. Then there was my grandmother, an attendant on her chest.

"What else can you do?"

I thought to call Henry but he'd be sleeping. The bleeding had eased. "I'll call Beth. I'm all right. Thank you. I'll be all right." With my head tilted back and the washcloth covering the lower half of my face, an old-fashioned bandit, I begged off and returned to my room.

Holy shit, I'd left the candle burning and damped it quickly before Nancy found out. Even with my truth told and my face smashed, I thought to hide the reality of the situation, to minimize the severity of my nightly fear.

I reached Beth, who was always up early with her kids. She'd been teaching nursery school but said she'd get a sub and be over to help me as soon as she was able. In the meantime, she instructed me to call her family physician, Dr. Borecky, who was an internist and cardiologist with a specialty in alcoholism. Maybe I wouldn't need the ER. But it was too early. His service took a message. I sat on my big-girl bed and wept.

Nancy had left me to it. Barbara Cook's version of "I Love the Piano" blared from her room. It was surreal. But then, nothing beat my self-flagellation. Of course I'd freaked her out. The time it took to receive the doctor's return call dragged on. Surely I would be committed.

Nancy appeared in my doorway, "Can I do anything?"

"Yes," I heard myself whisper, as if from far away, "you can sit by me until the doctor calls . . . please." And she did.

AFTER THE FALL

D r. Borecky was a middle-aged ginger with a nutty professor look. His practice was associated with St. Luke's-Roosevelt and his office was across the street from the hospital. He saw me immediately. His sense of urgency unnerved me. I kept waiting for him to announce that he would admit me for psychiatric care. At first, I didn't mention group therapy. I'd stuck to the facts of the incident. They were incriminating enough. But it was new territory sitting on that exam table. The brawl with myself had knocked the wind out of me. I could not locate my lies. I found myself telling him the truth about the night terrors and sleepwalking, how I'd had them since adolescence, had read about them as a teenager in *Psychology Today,* and had tolerated them as best I could.

The good doctor listened as he gently examined me. His total attention and his red hair reminded of Michael. He clucked his tongue and nodded his head. His concern was contagious. My resistance was down and I caught it. He held a hand mirror to my face and pointed to my upper lip to show me how my bottom tooth had pierced it when I'd hit the floor. I would need to see an oral surgeon immediately to examine my teeth and stitch my upper lip, if it required stitching. Because it was my face and I was an actress, he didn't want to do it himself. Both my top front teeth and one bottom tooth had been impacted and one was precariously loose. I also had a slight concussion.

He took blood to be sure no illness other than somnambulism had its hand in the accident. I asked for the mirror and dared to look again. My face was quite swollen by this point and I could not bite my lip to stop the tears. I'd always defined my worth by my beauty; appearances were of the utmost importance. As a kid, my looks had pleased my parents and made me feel loved.

He'd finished taking blood and handed me a box of tissues.

"I have an audition with a really good theatrical agent this week . . . I guess I'll have to postpone it now." My shoulders shook. It had been the first meeting of this caliber since I'd drank away my opportunities after graduating theatre school.

"Don't worry, your nose is fractured but not displaced. We'll have to wait a few weeks until the swelling recedes but I don't think you'll need surgery."

I nodded gratefully.

"We bleed a lot with injuries to our mouth and nose . . . I'm concerned about the cause, Miss Frazier. I'm concerned about the night terrors and sleepwalking. The accident could have been much worse."

The fluorescent office lights intensified my headache. I closed my eyes and saw my old neighbor's lonely corpse. Every inch of me ached, including my stomach. I'd been sucker punched by the new bed. It had been a setup and it was me who'd thrown the fight.

"You have to see Dr. Kavey up at Columbia's Sleep Clinic. He's the expert."

"I don't have insurance." I felt ten years old with my legs dangling from the table as another wave of tears threatened.

"Well, first we need to get you fixed up. In a couple of days, you'll come back and we'll have a long talk."

I cried harder but this time from relief. The threat of being committed receded. Dr. Borecky had heard me. He'd gotten it. He was gravely concerned, unlike the doctor I'd confided in as a teen who suggested I had "girly trouble" and told me to talk with my mother. He passed me the tissues again. I wanted to give my nose a good blow but couldn't. I patted my face so carefully, I smiled.

"You're going to be all right," he smiled back. "We'll get you up to see Dr. Kavey."

My front teeth didn't have to be pulled. The oral surgeon said I might need a root canal. We'd have to wait and see the damage. And I didn't need stiches. The scar would be minor and disappear into the outline of my upper lip.

I canceled my audition with the top theatrical agent due to the injuries to my face and it broke my heart. I told him I was unwell and that it might be some time before I contacted him again. As I hung up the phone, I wished I'd lied and said that there'd been a death in my family. It was clear he wouldn't take my future calls. I was a good actress but had not concealed my wavering voice. To invent a more glamorous excuse would have precipitated my dangerous denial and I knew it. The fall had broken more than my nose; it had broken my façade.

I holed up at Beth's house, grieved, and let her family love me. In the meantime, she, her husband, and some friends baby-proofed my room. They removed the box spring and left the mattress. They put away all glass, breakable or sharp objects, and moved one dresser in front of the window. They cleared any furniture from the area near the wall with the light switch so at least my path would be clear in case I made a run for it again.

A few days later, I met again with Dr. Borecky. He asked me extensively about my sleepwalking history. I left out the night of the open window. He asked about my family's sleep history, too, and pushed me to see the connection more definitively between growing up with alcoholism and the night terrors. I bragged about my dad's long-term sobriety, but when it came out that he'd been addicted to sleeping pills, Dr. Borecky said that my father hadn't been sober all those years—that his abuse of sleeping pills had constituted a slip. He was the expert on alcoholism but his insistence on that point bothered me tremendously. I couldn't keep up with my breaking denial.

Dr. Borecky practically begged me to see Dr. Kavey, but I didn't have hundreds of dollars to pay out of pocket. I had no savings. I couldn't see how it would be possible. His fee was quite high because it included an initial consultation, two nights of sleep study, and a follow-up visit. But the day after my second visit with Borecky, a good friend told me about an opening at the private school where she taught music. Their drama teacher was going on sabbatical for a year. I'd be able to interview within a few weeks. Hopefully my face would be healed. If I got it, I'd have medical insurance starting in September and would then be able to go to Columbia's Sleep Clinic.

A week after the accident, I was back to the scene of the crime. Sitting alone on my mattress, thawing from shock, I didn't think I would be able to sleep there ever again. I was deeply grateful to Beth and her family but they couldn't babysit me forever.

Henry and I spoke several times that Saturday. With each call, the sound of his cooing voice and his chorus of chirping birds calmed me. He'd been urging me to get out and attend a party. It was the last thing I wanted to do, but as evening approached, I couldn't stay put. Reluctantly, I moped along. I'd attempted to cover the bruises with makeup but felt excruciatingly vulnerable.

It was a big gathering with a DJ and I mostly hid in a corner. I wasn't planning to stay long. As I was preparing to leave, a tall, handsome man asked me to dance. I almost said no. I thought Mark was too good-looking and decided that he'd be full of himself. But a kindness shone from his dark eyes. I was both unnerved and attracted. We danced and then escaped the noise of the crowd and talked for hours in a quiet hallway, like teenagers.

In those early moments, while basking in the warmth of Mark's attention, I was reminded of the hours spent sharing from my heart with Michael Hoffman. I felt alternately desirous of this man's interest and damaged beyond repair. I was grateful that the corner we'd found was poorly lit and evaded his questions about my bruised face. He must have sensed there was a story I was afraid to tell. I was relieved that Mark asked for my number when the party ended. I hoped he would call.

A week after my fall, a friend recommended a psychologist who purportedly knew a lot about sleep and whose fee I could afford. I was terrified of another accident and couldn't wait to see Kavey. The psychologist suggested I see his associate, a psychiatrist who could prescribe an antidepressant to inhibit my dreams, which might prevent the somnambulism.

Might didn't sound promising. I was terrified of taking medicine. My father's sleeping pills had been prescribed but that hadn't stopped him from becoming addicted. Still, I needed a stop-gap measure. I took the referral, took extra shifts at the restaurant, and saw the psychologist's friend.

He was meticulously dressed, an A-type personality, young and preppy. He sat behind a desk and took notes. It wasn't a big desk but he was remote, miles away. When I asked him to recommend articles about my sleep disorders, he said I would not understand the medical literature. I hated his smugness. A parade of smug psychiatrists who'd cared for Billy stood behind him, so many boys whistling in the dark. I took the three-month prescription for the antidepressant he handed me. I was desperate. Just before we parted, he asked if there was anything else.

"Yes," I eked my way toward finding my voice, "you could appreciate the fact that I've stayed sober through all of this. That as a recovering alcoholic, I didn't slip and add that calamity to the fall."

"Oh, no," he quickly relented, "you're right."

It was as forthcoming as he could be, which was fine with me. I didn't care about being right. I wasn't fishing for compliments. I'd spoken up on my own behalf and that was good enough for me. I waved the prescription in appreciation and practically soared out of his office.

I nervously, very nervously, started on the antidepressant. Maybe it would tamper episodes enough to prevent an accident—until I, hopefully, scraped together the money to see Dr. Kavey.

A few days after the visit with the psychiatrist, I found the Center for Medical Consumers, by Washington Square Park in the Village, which was free and open to the public. There were very few articles on sleepwalking but several on night terrors and I read them all. I kept coming up against the term *post-traumatic stress disorder.* PTSD was prevalent among survivors of war, including veterans, as well as people who had experienced childhood violence or sexual assault. *Flashbacks,* *dissociation,* and *hyperarousal* were words that kept appearing and sent me back to the librarian with requests for further information.

As I pored over the medical research, my body was overcome with relief. My stomach unclenched and my shoulders relaxed. I was not alone. I felt empathy for my fellow sufferers. My heart softened toward myself. I suddenly felt my exhaustion, twenty years' worth. It was a rainy day and the place was quiet except for the hum of lights. Alone at my table, I rested my head on my arms and thought about my mother as a girl finding refuge in the Albany Public Library. I closed my eyes and fell asleep.

"Time to close, sweetheart," an older librarian gently shook my arm and startled me awake. Drool pooled on the table. Embarrassed, I wiped it away with my sleeve.

"I'm so sorry." My face was healing fast, but was still bruised. People's pitying glances unnerved me. I knew what they were thinking.

She had assisted me earlier and, whispered, "No reason to be sorry," and then, pointing to an article on PTSD, "that'll knock you out cold."

We smiled. Her kindness touched me. She was transgender, and I wondered at all we go through in becoming ourselves.

I took the rush hour subway home and got a seat wedged between two suits. Despite it being packed, the commuter sitting next to me nodded off. His head bobbed awfully close to my shoulder. When I was drinking, I'd pass out on the train. Now I hated the idea of falling asleep in public. Thank goodness the librarian had been kind. I hoped the librarians had been kind to my mother when she'd dozed off in the stacks as a girl. The thick knot of my family's stories seized my stomach but since my sleepwalking accident, I'd skipped group therapy. It was on that ride home that I realized I wouldn't return. I knew one-on-one treatment was in order. I simply couldn't untangle this mess in a crowd. Even riding the subway unnerved me. My denial about the PTSD further shattered. I was surprised the racket didn't wake my napping neighbor.

I began interviewing individual therapists. I was determined to find a savvy, empathetic person to help me untangle the traumas that had stalked my sleep. I also wrote Dr. Smug and informed him about the Center for Medical Consumers in case another stupid layperson ever asked him for help in understanding an illness.

All of this transpired in the first few weeks after the sleepwalking accident. Something had irrevocably changed since my fall, since seeing Dr. Borecky, and since my visit to the medical library. I was still having episodes despite the antidepressant and longed to recover. I feared I might not survive the next fight.

Meanwhile, Mark and I had enjoyed a couple of rendezvous. He was the best kisser I'd ever met, almost as though he were trying to kiss me awake. Each encounter ended with my making some excuse and a quick departure. Finally, on date three, in the middle of another languid make-out session on the couch in his Chelsea apartment, I kissed him with tender lips still swollen from the fall. He gently traced the outline of my mouth and whispered, "What really happened here?"

"Like I said, you should have seen the other guy." This time he stared at me with concern in his dark eyes, encouraging me to say more.

"I've got an early day tomorrow. I should go." I stood up but he caught my wrist playfully and pulled me back to his lap.

"Not tonight." He cupped my face in his hands. "Why won't you stay with me?"

It was a good question. He was a thirty-three-year-old businessman—dreamy, smart, available, and interested. "You want me to pay this idiot a visit?" He pointed to the fading bruises on my face.

I felt trapped. I might lose this great guy if I told him the truth. I might lose him if I didn't. Tears spilled against my will. I wiped them away but Mark comforted me, and the storm passed. We sat on the couch, facing each other, awkwardly holding hands. I could tell by his pitying look he still thought I was in denial about an abusive man. I knew how easy it would be to let him believe that. Still, it wouldn't solve my problem—my fear of staying the night.

I wanted to go to bed with him and to sleep with him.

I took a breath and confessed, "Nobody did this to me, Mark. I did it to myself . . . I'm a sleepwalker. It's . . . serious. I had an accident."

Maybe growing up the oldest of eight children had cultivated Mark's sensitivity. Maybe the death of his sister when he was twelve had nurtured his empathy because all he said was, "Do you want to tell me about it?" Then he put his arm around me. For a few moments, we just sat side by side. It was a relief not to be looking directly into his face. He stroked my hair. I closed my eyes. I was tired all the time.

I recalled my father's definition of surrender—to join the winning side.

Mark held me through the night as I told him my story. When morning broke, he dragged the mattress from his bed and we slept together, soundly.

WINKIN, BLINKIN, AND NOD

By June, I landed the teaching job at the private school to start in September. I scheduled an appointment with Dr. Kavey for the fall. Knowing it was in place gave me great relief. My physical injuries healed and I found a wonderful therapist, Neila Wyman, who worked on a sliding scale through the Gestalt Institute.

Mark and I became serious. He was recently separated and shared custody of his son, who was two years old. As we were getting to know each other, we only dated every other weekend when Zachary was with his mom. We wanted time as a couple before the three of us started hanging out. Still, Mark's parenting affected me.

I did have episodes, and he met them with sensitivity and patience. One night we lay on his mattress—he'd donated the rest of his bed to Goodwill—I was having trouble falling asleep and we told each other the stories of our day. Zach had thrown a tantrum. He'd been exhausted and had flung himself flat out on the sidewalk on the corner of Ninety-Sixth and Broadway, crying miserably.

"What did you do?" I asked, expecting him to say he'd lost control and spanked Zach or yelled at him in front of the crowd that had stopped to gawk.

"I picked him up and held him."

"You're treating him like a baby," I blurted.

Mark paused and looked sadly at me, "Kathleen . . . he is a baby."

I burst into tears of apology and shame. Mark gave me the same reproach he'd given Zach. He held me heart-to-heart. Soon mine calmed to his steady beat and I got it, in that moment, how I'd been calloused—raised on rough. I was thirty and an old dog. I worried that I was too far gone to learn new tricks.

Toward the end of the summer, Nancy asked me to move out. She claimed she needed the apartment to herself, but I believed it was because of the accident. I didn't blame her. I had a friend in the neighborhood, Maureen, who owned a beautiful apartment on West End Avenue and was looking to rent out the maid's room behind her kitchen. I'd have my own bathroom and shower. Mark helped me haul my few belongings through the neighborhood and unpack.

When it came time for him to leave, a sadness came over me. Maybe I would always be somebody's roommate—a renter, one step away from homeless. He insisted that I spend the night at his place. Instead of pretending everything was okay and white-knuckling my feelings, I agreed.

It was oppressively hot. I woke drenched in sweat and in a panic, unsure if I'd had an episode. I'd startled Mark awake and he held me. I felt awful. I was a freak. How much more of this nonsense could he stand before he broke it off?

"I'm sorry," I tried to pull away.

"No," he said, "don't do that"—the very words Michael had said all those years ago on the night of the storm when I'd had to leave him. Back then, I couldn't utter one word about the sleepwalking or the depths of my fear of losing him.

"Don't leave," Mark whispered, "I got you."

I was undone. My terror and self-hatred unleashed. I let myself have the tantrum I'd been suppressing all those thousands of nights. Unlike when I was a toddler, wailing for comfort from my crib, he didn't leave me alone. He listened silently to my tirade. He held the space for me like it was nothing to him. He witnessed my self-loathing and he didn't flinch.

When I'd run out of steam, Mark firmly ordered me to give him my hand. As I did, it recalled the slapping game Danny and I'd played as kids. I braced myself for the blow. I deserved it. It was love to me. Instead, my boyfriend gently stroked my hand. He patted and kissed it. Again I dissolved into tears and he held me close.

Just as I was becoming willing to truly face and release the illness that had stolen twenty years of sleep and left my face battered, just as I was becoming willing to release the self-violence and seek proper help, I'd met this man who modeled gentle love. I thought of Henry whispering in my ear at Happy Burger, "Let us love you until you learn to love yourself."

September finally arrived. I stepped out of the subway at 168th Street in Washington Heights and was struck with the desire to turn my back on Columbia-Presbyterian, run down Broadway through Harlem until I reached the Upper West Side, and lock myself away in my little, old maid's room.

Dr. Kavey was dark haired and dark eyed with wire-rimmed glasses. Small of stature and wiry, he sat behind an imposing wooden desk. My heart thumped, no first impressions, only dread. What if he turned out to be another Dr. Smug? Images of accompanying my mother on all those consultations when Billy was sick sat behind me, like so many monkeys on my back. He sensed my nervousness and poured me some water. I didn't touch the glass for fear of spilling it all over myself, or worse, all over his beautiful desk.

"Dr. Borecky says you've got quite a story. Why don't you tell me about yourself?"

He smiled and I felt my shoulders relax. He appreciated all I'd been though as well as the research I'd done on my own behalf. It was the first time I'd met someone who really understood my sleep disorders and the havoc they'd wreaked on my life. I confided about how I'd self-medicated with alcohol and was sober five years.

"Good for you. No easy task, that."

He'd passed my litmus test effortlessly. I told him I'd known about my sleep disorders since I was sixteen, from the *Psychology Today* article, and that I felt bad for not finding help sooner.

"Well don't feel bad. Most sleepwalkers don't seek help until they hurt themselves or somebody else. The shame and denial are just that strong. When that article was written in 1975, there were only three sleep clinics in the whole country. Now there are more than a hundred and fifty. We've come a long way, even while our understanding of sleep is still in its infancy."

"I've always been afraid of being misdiagnosed. I have a brother who's schizophrenic. I've held my breath my whole life for fear of being institutionalized, carted away in the middle of a somnambulant episode." My eyes filled and Dr. Kavey passed me a box of tissues.

"People with sleep disorders are misdiagnosed all the time, all kinds of misdiagnoses. I heard a narcoleptic speak recently at a conference. She'd been scheduled for brain surgery until, luckily, a hospital resident recognized her symptoms during a preliminary procedure."

He paused, then asked, "How's your brother doing?"

It moved me, him asking after Billy. We talked about my brother's incredible fortitude in the face of his illness, about his suicide attempts so long ago, and how my sleepwalking had taken on the added component of night terrors when he'd first taken ill.

I explained that my remembered episodes were almost always accompanied by an urgency to escape whomever or whatever was coming to get me. I inquired about night terrors as a symptom of post-traumatic stress disorder. He said that most patients do not report a history of trauma. In the next breath, he supported my efforts toward emotional health and seconded my decision to continue therapy.

"It's not uncommon for parasomnias to run in families although we haven't figured out the genetic link."

A genetic link made sense. I also wondered if sleepwalking runs in families as a learned effect or symptom of the pattern of trauma that can repeat intergenerationally—if it was like alcoholism in that way. Did a person become an alcoholic or were they born one? Was I predisposed to night terrors? If everyone who experienced trauma sleepwalked then there'd be a lot more sleepwalking going on. Although, considering how I'd gone to such lengths to hide my malady, maybe there were plenty more somnambulists secreting-away their violent episodes?

Dr. Kavey said parasomnias are sometimes called disorders of arousal because something breaks through, triggers them. Researchers don't know what exactly; in some cases, it's noise. Sleepers are propelled from deep, quiet non-REM sleep into partial wakefulness without going through the usual stages.

I told him I'd read about the term *arousal disorders*.

"It's a pretty mild term for what, in sleepers like you, can impel you to have sustained such critical physical injuries."

I let my tears flow freely then.

"I am truly sorry for all you've had to endure, Miss Frazier. We can help you. I am confident that we'll have you sleeping soundly."

Sleeping soundly—I wanted to believe Dr. Kavey, but it seemed impossible. I acted as if it were, though, and followed his instructions. He asked me to keep a sleep journal for a week prior to my evaluation. I recorded when I took naps, how many hours I slept each night, and any episodes that I could recall. He'd told me to stop the antidepressant. It would be important to the analysis of my sleep patterns that my two nights at the center be as typical as possible.

He had said that the episodes create abnormally intense brain activity resembling a seizure on an EEG. He expected to prescribe a miniscule dose of Klonopin as an anticonvulsant. Antidepressants suppress REM sleep, while night terrors, unlike nightmares, occur in non-REM sleep.

Dr. Borecky adamantly warned me against the 0.25 milligrams per night of Klonopin that Dr. Kavey was expecting to prescribe after the study. It's in the benzodiazepine family and often prescribed in much higher doses as an anti-anxiety and panic disorder medication. Valium, Xanax, Ativan, and Dalmane are all benzodiazepines. Borecky worried that even though it would be a small dosage of Klonopin, it could lead to abuse, especially with my history of alcoholism. Now I was afraid I would repeat my father's ordeal and become addicted to the very medicine that was supposed to cure my sleep problem.

Dr. Kavey called me a few days before my study. He had talked to Borecky and was concerned I was chickening out. He assured me that the Klonopin was a stop-gap measure, that at such a low dosage and with close monitoring, I would be fine. *Stop-gap*, isn't that what Dr. Smug's antidepressant, which hadn't worked anyway, was supposed to be?

He cautioned me not to put the cart before the horse, to have the study, and he'd talk with Dr. Borecky again before we made a plan.

I pushed, "Dr. Borecky said that even if I didn't misuse the Klonopin that withdrawal is dangerous and can actually cause seizures."

"That's if it's stopped abruptly. I can't emphasize enough what a low dose you'll be on, Miss Frazier, and how you and I will see each other regularly. And when you're ready to stop the Klonopin, we'll decrease it very, very slowly."

"If it's so small to begin with, how will we decrease it?"

"Instead of taking the 0.25 milligrams every night, we'll have you skip a night for a while and then another and another. Incrementally, the nights without the Klonopin will increase. I can assure you, my patients have had tremendous success on this medicine."

Dr. Kavey had called me for another reason besides a pep talk about his expected course of treatment. He'd been approached by *Vogue* for an article on sleep disorders. In addition to interviewing him, they hoped to interview one of his patients and he asked me if I'd be willing. They wouldn't use my name, only the initial K.

"I guess so, if you think it will help other sleepwalkers."

"I do," he said.

A long pause followed. I felt my mother at my side, and her mother standing beside her, and on and on, shoulder to shoulder, backward through time. Maybe many had suffered from sleepwalking and night terrors, or I'd only imagined them that way. I had to speak up, anyway I could.

"Okay," I peeped.

The reporter would meet me at the clinic on the second night of my study.

I'd been missing my mom terribly after the accident and especially as I prepared for the sleep study. The night before my stay at the clinic, I dreamt of her.

In the dream we were sitting together, just the two of us, in a glass room on the top floor of a tall building. A wintry landscape spread below us, as far as the eye could see. Even the sky was pale. We sat across from each other at a small, wooden table holding hands and admiring the view. Suddenly, the most beautiful snowy white owl flew by, so close we could have touched her except for the window.

"Wow, Mom, can you imagine being able to fly?"

"Yes," and she gazed directly into my eyes.

In that moment, I knew that I would be free of the sleepwalking someday.

I weathered the first night at the clinic with no episodes. I felt both relieved and worried. What if Dr. Kavey thought I'd been making up stories of sleepwalking? What if he diagnosed me with Munchausen syndrome and sentenced me to the New York Psychiatric Institute, which was right around the corner from Columbia-Presbyterian's Sleep Center?

I had the day between studies off from teaching. Henry was dying and I visited him. I'd been putting it off. If I didn't see him maybe he wouldn't leave me, but the moment we were together my heart lifted and my mind eased. He was conscious and serene. He'd found shelter for his many birds. It had been his main worry, that they'd be left unattended.

I held the Birdman's delicate hand. "You saved my life, Henry."

"You saved mine. That's how it works. We save each other."

"You've been like a mother to me." We laughed because he could be a bit of a nag when he'd worried about me over the years and I'd often begged him to stop mothering me.

I told him about my mother's visitation the other night.

"Wow," he clucked his tongue, "snowy white owls . . . they defend their young fiercely."

"So, I guess she's helping me through this mess." I didn't sound too convinced.

"She's always with you. She told you that herself, right?"

I nodded and kissed his hand, knowing he was talking about himself too.

"Tell me more about the owl." It pleased him, to show off about his birds and it might prevent my threatening tears, my obsession to make everything about me.

"Well, the obvious . . . wisdom, intuition, the ability to see what others do not see . . . change . . . death."

Henry held my gaze for a long, loving moment and I didn't falter.

"Big change . . ." he added, "maybe it's time you stop having night terrors and start having visions."

I smiled but Henry was serious. He was part Choctaw. I was awed by his depth of understanding regarding all things spiritual, which were all things to him.

"Snowy white owl . . . you've got yourself a powerful totem."

That night was cold for September as I ventured to Washington Heights with my overnight bag for the second part of the study. The winds picked up as I turned a corner toward the clinic. A storm was coming, and I hoped the winds would blow away my old life and make room for the new. Mark had offered to escort me as he had the first night but I understood this was my odyssey—to be faced alone.

Rachel Urquhart, the reporter from *Vogue*, met me at the sleep clinic. She was young and watched with a journalist's eye as Joe, the medical technician, attached twenty-five electrodes to my head and body. Most were affixed to my head to monitor my brain and eye activity.

"You look like Medusa," Rachel teased.

Joe laughed and I did, too. He looked about fourteen, especially as he giggled, but had assured me he was in his twenties. The whole scene was surreal, especially knowing my story would be published. I was grateful to be anonymous and couldn't have allowed the interview otherwise. I'd recently experimented with telling a coworker that I had a sleep disorder. "Don't use that term," he'd warned as he circled his forefinger toward his head in the universal sign for cracked. "It sounds like you're crazy."

Dr. Kavey called after the last electrode was applied and instructed me to have a restless but comfortable night. "Now I have performance anxiety," I joked as we hung up and my audience of two laughed. There was an awful lot of fooling around considering I felt like vomiting.

Rachel left before bedtime, and even though she was a stranger, I had that old familiar dread of her leaving me to it.

The faux bedroom had been decorated to be cozy but only left me feeling ridiculous. There was a television, a potted palm, a framed landscape poster, and a huge, stuffed Cookie Monster in a rocking chair. Old and worn, he seemed desperate for a glass of milk, a plate of cookies, and a good night's sleep. As a kid, I'd felt sorry for my stuffed animals because they couldn't close their eyes and rest. On the other hand, I hadn't wanted them to rest. They were my bodyguards.

Suddenly I felt repulsed by how gullible I'd been, duped into believing a toy or an angel, a dead relative or a dream-bird, had watched over me in the night. Joe would be stationed in the adjoining room in case a machine went haywire and needed immediate attention or in case *I* went haywire and needed immediate attention. But even a real, live guard could not protect me against my mind.

The second study was turning out to be much more difficult than the first. The visit to Henry had unnerved me. The interview had undone me.

I shook as I climbed into the hospital bed from the bottom. One side faced a wall and a metal guardrail was in place at the other. Joe turned the overhead fluorescents off and the night-light on, but not before I gave a stoic wave into the camera that hung above the bed to record my every toss and turn.

"You're funny," he said as I lay down.

"I know, right?" and as he closed the door, I wiped away my tears with the back of my hand surreptitiously, in hopes the camera wouldn't catch it.

Stoic comes from the Greek word *stoa*, as in "colonnade," or stone pillar.

There was no way to find comfort with more than two dozen electrodes stuck to me. The night before I'd hardly slept but must have been in denial about how uncomfortable the whole process was. This night I was angered by the wires and adhesive. I felt like a human guinea pig. Those electrodes fixed to my head were the worst. Rachel had been right: sleepwalking had cursed me and turned me into a hideous monster— Medusa with reptiles for hair. I could never reconcile that Athena had punished the beautiful maiden for being raped by Poseidon—how the girl had paid for his violence. After the curse, those who looked at her were turned into stone. Even after her head had been cut off and placed on Athena's shield, she continued to petrify her victims.

I closed my eyes and the snake terror from my teens, the one that had sent me flying down the stairs, flashed before me. I startled and called out to Joe, "Don't worry, that wasn't a night terror. I'm just nervous."

He peeked his head in. "Everyone we hook up is nervous. I don't know how anybody sleeps with all those attachments. Can I get you a sip of water?"

"No thanks, Joe. I'm fine."

I realized my hand was outstretched in a *go away* pose. I couldn't even stand the technician who was *supposed* to see me this way seeing me this way. Lying in the hotbed of science, armed to the hilt with all the medical information known to mankind about somnambulism, I felt cursed. With Henry's spiritual pep talk still ringing in my ears, I felt repugnant. Mark's gentle face came to mind but my heart turned rock-hard, like in the old days.

How easy it had been to leave Don; how relieved I'd felt when Theo took up with the actor's daughter, and then there was Michael's pained look on the night of the storm when I'd had to go. My new boyfriend seemed determined to love me, but would I be able to break this sleepwalking spell and love him in return? I hadn't turned the men who'd gazed at me into stone, but I had hardened my own heart. Was I even capable of love, of change, as my snowy owl totem suggested? Or had Henry's interpretation of my dream been just an old man's ranting, concocted to save himself from the ultimate terror?

It was almost funny in its predictability, my fear of death, my fear of living. Lying in that hospital bed hooked up to machines with red lights flashing and my heart beating its petrified beat, I fully realized that the men in my life had been a smoke screen for the real question: could I face myself? Could I look myself in the eyes and love myself, electrodes and all?

About a week later, I sat opposite Dr. Kavey at his beautiful desk for my follow-up visit. The twelve EEG pens had scrawled over two thousand pages during my two nights' study in response to the electrodes. The machines had monitored and measured my heart rates, brain and eye activity, breathing, muscle tension, and leg movements.

I had not had a night terror or sleepwalking episode either evening and found myself apologizing.

"Well," he replied, "somebody here recently had a very severe accident."

I thought he was referring to some other patient who'd recently stayed at the clinic. That's how strong my denial still was.

"I'm sorry to hear that." As I spoke, my stomach sank for the sleepwalking stranger. "I hope they weren't hurt badly."

Dr. Kavey gave me an incredulous look.

"Kathleen, I was referring to you. You had a severe accident from sleepwalking and night terrors." And then he said three words that changed my life forever—

"You suffered enough."

VISIONS OF BABY'S BREATH

I started on the Klonopin and began sleeping the night through for the first time in twenty years. Twenty years is a long time without good shut-eye—about 7,500 nights and two-thirds of my life. I felt joyful, saved. At the same time, I was unprepared for the deep well of grief. I waded through with the help of those near and dear. I mourned with Neila in therapy and, come nightfall, in Mark's arms.

There was a Volkswagen commercial when I was a kid, a gag where person after person climbed out of the tiny car. My body was that car and the people were traumas stored. Slowly, I unpacked the baggage I'd lugged from night to night—from year to year. Gently, my therapist held a safe space for me to have my feelings while wide awake, instead of acting them out while sleepwalking. Gestalt was ideal. The techniques went beyond talk therapy and engaged all of me— body, mind, and spirit. I understood the importance of releasing the traumas from my body. If I learned one thing from all that nocturnal wandering, it's that the body doesn't lie.

Fear of abusing the medication loomed while I struggled to believe what Dr. Kavey had said, *You suffered enough*. My denial kept creeping in and this is what it told me: you haven't suffered traumatic events cataclysmic enough to cause PTSD, to cause sleep terrors, and you are making all this up—*you are a liar*. Neila pointed out that from there, it was less than one giant step to *you'd better not say what goes on in this house* and *Kathy's so quiet you wouldn't even know she was here.*

This was the early 1990s when the term False Memory Syndrome (FMS) was coined to describe a condition in which a person's identity and relationships are affected by memories that are factually incorrect but that they strongly believe. Neila spent a lot of time assuring me that I didn't have FMS, that the facts of my life, of my days and of my nights, were enough. I had suffered enough.

I hung up my gloves and surrendered. Once again, I joined the winning side—one, nightly 0.25 milligram dosage of Klonopin at a time—one weekly therapy session at a time.

Eventually Mark and I moved in together. Eventually we bought a bed. He slept on the outside and I slept against the wall. Bedtime rituals included a moratorium on worrisome topics, lots of hugs, and the donning of what Mark calls my "get-up"—earplugs and an eye mask to decrease the possibility of being startled into an episode.

I continued to benefit from witnessing my boyfriend's healthy parenting of Zach. From them, I learned the link between comfort, trust, and peaceful slumber. Going to bed became about rituals, about winding down, reading fluff, about praying and comforting the little girl in me, about calming the teenager in me, about celebrating the woman in me.

I did sometimes have disturbed sleep, for example, if I'd seen a violent scene in a movie.

One winter's day, I witnessed a parent's cruelty toward a boy on the street. I'd read that to intervene would only make it worse for the child. Cold winds had driven most everybody indoors and it was icy underfoot. He was about five and had dropped his toy while crossing Broadway. She scurried with the slumped shoulders of exhaustion. When they reached the curb, he realized his loss and started crying. She grabbed him by the shoulders and let him have it. Shake, shake, shake. Then one, two, three wallops hard on his behind. He was a little thing. He slipped and fell to the sidewalk. The berating started as she dragged him to his feet by his arm.

She was only spanking him, a little too hard, but it was her God-given American right, right? Spare the rod and spoil the child? Standing nearby, frozen with fear and powerlessness, I felt every blow. I closed my eyes and prayed, DON'T . . . GIVE . . . UP.

That night I screamed and sat bolt upright in bed, heart racing. Mark sat up, too, almost simultaneously, and held me. It was as though he'd entered my sleep terror, lying there beside me, only to emerge when I had, his embrace at the ready. I came to quickly and worried—had I awakened Zach in the next room?

Mark checked him and reported back, "No worries, he sleeps like the dead," but the common analogy walloped me like the mother had walloped the boy that bitter day. This is what I realized—when you're a little thing and the person you look up to hits you or berates you, or if they do the same to someone you love, you grow to both fear death and to long for it.

Mark held me tenderly as I recounted the scene on the sidewalk. "I'm falling apart," I fretted between sobs.

"You're not falling apart. You're falling together." My head was to his chest and he hummed. He was shy to sing but had this way of rumbling low that combined with the steady beat of his heart. It calmed me quickly. Then he massaged my feet with oil and placed them in woolen socks from Ireland. "I heard that helps a person sleep."

"I like it that they're Irish," and we smiled.

Mark hates reading aloud, but will comply if I beg. He read me my favorite poem of Margaret Atwood's—"Variations on the Word Sleep." It describes perfectly a longing to enter sleep with your beloved as its smooth, dark wave slides over her head and to protect her from her worst fear and from the grief at the center of her dream.

I understood that Mark could not accompany me into sleep or protect me from my fears and grief. I knew he could not usher me safely from that watery underworld back into my worried body. With time, however, I'd grown certain that he would be there to greet me when each new day broke and that together we would embrace the intimacy that for years I had fled.

Many things became clear to me as time went on; I noticed that sometimes a mild sleep terror episode would coincide with the onset of my menstrual cycle. Dr. Kavey and I decided to raise the 0.25 milligrams of Klonopin to 0.50 each month for just a few nights before my period. He'd kept his promise and we had follow-up visits regularly. So far, I had not stepped out of bed. So far, I had not abused the medicine.

The intersections between my hormonal cycle, sleep, creativity, and intuition fascinated me. I remembered my dreams more frequently, wrote them down, and shared them in therapy. My acting work, especially at The Actors Studio, blossomed and finally made real sense to me.

I was thirty-five when Mark and I married and had spent five years on the Klonopin. It had been fifteen years after my failed marriage with Don, which felt like a lifetime ago. I was a different person, steeped in my search for health, and finally able to offer true partnership. We wanted to have a baby but taking the medication during pregnancy could cause birth defects. I began to decrease the dosage under Dr. Kavey's supervision. Worry escalated—maybe violent episodes would return. Mark and I'd decided that if they did, I would go back on the medicine and we'd consider adoption.

My deep, deep desire to have a child with Mark made me willing to go to any lengths to prevent a sleepwalking relapse. Dr. Kavey had suggested morning walks to set my internal clock and to, as much as possible, keep a regular bedtime. He also encouraged me to nap if I slept poorly. Sleep specialists usually discourage insomniacs from napping, but sleepwalking and sleep terrors commonly escalate with lack of sleep. I practiced meditation and received acupuncture to quiet my nerves. I saw a hypnotherapist who taught me techniques not unlike meditation toward calming myself at bedtime or if I woke panicked in the night. I still sometimes had insomnia at the times when I used to sleepwalk, around 1:00 and 4:00 a.m.

I worked with a nutritionist, Annie Fox, who was an RN, a homeopath, and an herbalist. She once treated a woman who used to cook and eat whole meals while sleepwalking. Annie had very strong opinions about the effects of low blood sugar. From her experience, it was often associated with alcoholics and sleepwalkers. Like my father, I am hypoglycemic. I have low blood pressure and tend toward anemia. She said my habit of eating sugary cereal in an effort to calm and ground myself after episodes or even during middle-of-the-night bouts of insomnia proved the phenomenon of craving. She explained that the best way to stop my body's need for sugar and white flour in the night was to give them up altogether—that it would mean less chance of a recurrence of somnambulism if I did so.

I stopped eating sugar. I hadn't had coffee in years and gave up the occasional, treasured cup of decaf coffee and Earl Grey tea. I could not deny the positive effects of iron, magnesium, and vitamin B rich foods in my diet and also began a regime of vitamins and supplements.

I noticed that if I skipped the B complex for an extended period of time, I had a minor night terror. The doctor who had helped my father kick the sleeping pills so many years ago had prescribed vitamin B shots as he detoxed.

Annie also suggested I give up dairy because I have a deviated septum, and she thought that quitting milk and cheese might help eliminate my snoring and help me sleep better. It proved harder than letting go of sweets but when tempted with a creamy Brie or robust blue, especially at parties, I'd imagine myself holding a swaddled pack of cheese like in *I Love Lucy* when Lucy tried to smuggle some dairy delicacies out of Italy on a plane. I'd think, *What do I want, a cheese-baby or a baby-baby?*

A baby-baby.

Henry had died soon after my stay at the sleep clinic. I missed my old friend and thought of him often, especially whenever I had a dream that was more of a vision—like the one with my mom and the snowy white owl.

One night, while coming off the Klonopin, I dreamt of what felt like an ancient time.

In the dream, it was the middle of the night in the middle of a forest clearing, surrounded by rolling hills covered in tall oaks. I was part of a procession of women, and each of us wore a long, white gown. We walked from the top of the knolls, down to a shimmering lake, a magical lake. A full moon illuminated our path and Ellen Burstyn stood nearby. She was the leader—a high priestess—and was pleased with the scene before her. One at a time, each woman reached into the mysterious waters of the so-still lake and pulled out her personal power or gift. My sister, Patricia, was before me and her hands surfaced strewn with gold, silver, and jewels. My turn came. I plunged my hands into the water, which was icy cold and sent a jolt of awareness through my dream-body. *I am awake now*, I dream-thought; *I am conscious*. My hands were full of living, growing things, beautiful vines, roses, leaves, and moss in the shape of a cross, but older than a Christian cross. It was primeval and palpitated in my open hands and gave them the power to heal.

In real life, Ellen Burstyn had continued to mentor and mother me. She'd officiated at our wedding and Mark, Zach, and I spent many holidays in her home. I consider her a spiritual advisor as well as an artistic one so her role in my dream made perfect sense. Plus I had recently re-watched one of my favorite films—*Resurrection*. In it, Ellen plays a woman who dies in a car crash, is resuscitated, and awakes to discover that she has become a healer.

We met for lunch at West Bank Café and I recounted my dream. I also confided about coming off the Klonopin and my trepidation over a possible relapse, how I longed to be free of the medicine and to conceive.

"You have to write about the sleepwalking and find a way to get it out into the world."

Terrifying—what could she possibly be thinking? "I'm not a writer. Besides, how can I write about what I hardly remember?"

"Start from what you know. Start from the acting. Use sense memory exercises to explore the bits and pieces you do recall. Lee used to say, *you'll be amazed what happens when you just make the effort.*"

Ellen was referring to Lee Strasberg, cofounder of The Group Theatre, which led to the creation of The Actors Studio. Originator of the acting technique known as the Method, he led the Studio for many years and had taught Ellen, as well as a long list of other brilliant stage and film actors. Strasberg died in 1982, a year before I first became a finalist, so I never met him but have learned tremendously from his disciples.

She smiled wisely. "Don't you see? It's the next right thing to do. It's our actors' alchemy . . . it's time to reach into that dark lake of your subconscious mind and transform all that suffering into art."

We were to dessert by this time and I felt I should have been more enthused by her inspirational speech. I dunked my chamomile tea bag nervously. It seemed like every effort was to calm myself and this idea of sharing my story in some public way riled me up inside. It was the antithesis of *Kathy's so quiet, you wouldn't even know she was here.* It was tantamount to putting Invisible Girl on stage, shining a magic spotlight, and revealing me for the freak I was.

"I'm ashamed to say, I'm afraid people will think I'm a freak." I lowered my voice as the hostess seated a couple at a nearby table.

Ellen laughed out loud and diners turned their heads, an excuse to take a long look at the famous actress. "We're all freaks, Kathleen. We've all been traumatized one way or another, each of us dissociated, a little or a lot . . . sleepwalking through life, bumbling our way toward consciousness. The only difference between the audience and the artists is that we have to do it . . . to save our lives . . . we're brave or dumb enough, depending on how you look at it, to screw our courage to the sticking post and bare our souls."

I put pen to paper, a nervous scrawl, supported by Ellen and three other Studio members—Vivian Nathan, Jacqueline Knapp, and Dina Janis. Dina spent hours gently leading me through Affective Memory exercises and directed me in my first reading at the Studio of a patchwork of pieces. Vivian moderated acting sessions where I also read passages. She'd been a member since the late 1940s and it was the first time she'd seen an actor write from sensory exercises. Jacqueline directed various incarnations of the work in progress at The Cornelia Street Café, one of the few remaining artists' haunts from the 1970s in Greenwich Village.

Even if they hadn't experienced sleepwalking, audiences found it fascinating. Many grew up with or knew a somnambulist. Like Ellen predicted, people overwhelmingly identified with the circumstances that had exacerbated my malady—growing up with alcoholism and mental illness and self-medicating with alcohol, other substances, or addictive behaviors. Everyone sleeps . . . or tries to, and most of us have struggled one way or another, at one time or another, with letting go into that mysterious realm. Then there was the uncharted territory of sleep and intimacy.

The more I wrote, the better I slept. Once again, my creative community had saved me. Word by word, the artistic process restored me. Turning my story into art proved transformative and led me to investigate further the relationship between sleepwalking and intuition. As a part of that exploration, Mark and I were invited to participate in open ceremonies led by First Nations people.

I felt Henry at my side during these gatherings and was amazed to learn about a special relationship between my ancestors and his. In the 1830s, the Choctaw tribe was forcibly removed from their ancestral home in Mississippi. They were marched in the middle of one of the coldest winters on record to what is now known as

Oklahoma—the first of many tribes to trudge the Trail of Tears. An estimated ten thousand died in the ethnic cleansing.

A decade later, the Choctaw people heard about the Potato Famine in Ireland. In 1847, they made a donation of $170 to the Irish Famine Relief, an amount equivalent to many thousands of dollars today.

I once heard a Choctaw man talk about his ancestors' donation. Someone asked what the reasoning had been behind such a generous gift from a people who had suffered overwhelming losses and who were themselves devastatingly poor. He said that his ancestors' generosity was because of those losses. It didn't matter that the famished strangers were far across the sea. To ignore the suffering of the Irish would have insulted their own relatives who had perished the same way. But when they gave freely, it not only fed the Irish but also the spirits of their Choctaw relatives who had died on the Trail of Tears.

We were outside in Central Park during this discussion on a blustery spring day, "Call it God or Great Spirit . . . benevolence goes by a thousand names around our Mother Earth," the Choctaw man concluded, "and to choose compassion . . . we save each other's lives."

Wind shook the trees when he said, *we save each other's lives*, and a host of sparrows soared skyward—Henry showing off.

By the end of May 1996, I'd been completely off the Klonopin for five months. So far, so good, and Dr. Kavey, along with my other health practitioners, cleared me to begin trying to conceive.

On June 21, Mark and I attended a solstice celebration at Breezy Point Beach in Brooklyn. I had no idea what to expect but was told we would mark the turning of the season, call in blessings for the summer, and have a lot of fun. Our friends knew about our hope to become pregnant. A number of them had recently been to Peru. When we arrived, Franklin Coursin, who is part Cherokee, excitedly put necklaces around our necks. They were made of red and black Huayruro seeds, symbols of fertility and abundance. "Now wait until y'all get home to start practicing," and he hooted while our faces turned as red as his gift.

Months earlier, I had purchased a tiny pair of handmade, beautifully beaded moccasins from Clyde Hall, a Shoshone friend. I had asked him to bless them and had placed them on our meditation altar at home. I'd been praying to be worthy to have them filled.

At Breezy Point, we were a group of about thirty people of all ages and races. We held hands, sang, and danced barefoot in the sand. The sun rose above the Atlantic as we rattled and drummed to a heartbeat rhythm. I felt silly and self-conscious but remembered a similar joy while twirling alone in the grass as a kid to the Beatles' "Fool on the Hill."

It had rained the night before and in the moment when I decided to let go of my self-consciousness, Mark squeezed my hand—*Look up,* he urged. We'd been singing a song about walking with beauty. In the sky above us appeared a double rainbow. We all oohed and aahed "Everything is connected!" our dear friend, Charles Lawrence, called out.

In that instant, I saw Grandma Frazier's weary face surrounded by her soft white hair that I'd loved to pat as a child. When she was a girl, she had fancied dancing at the crossroads in Ireland. I felt my grandparents at my side, and my mother, and Henry, and Michael too. I thought about my almitas' struggles and their kindnesses. I felt the kindnesses of so many dear ones who had beaconed my way through my dark night of the soul. Kindness—from the word *kin.*

Suddenly, I felt an overwhelming appreciation to my family for all they'd survived and for their heroic efforts toward health. My heart filled with emotion for my brothers and sisters, at how we'd tried to protect each other in whatever faltering ways we could while growing up. I felt love for my father and grateful for his sobriety. We'd become estranged after my sleepwalking accident but it wouldn't be long until we reconciled.

With my new friends at the beach, I let the wind crumble my stoicism to sand and then I wiggled my toes in it, boldly taking my pleasure. I held Mark's hand tighter, looked again at the double rainbow arching the Brooklyn sky, and knew I'd found the gold.

That evening of the summer solstice, Mark and I made love in our Washington Heights home overlooking the Hudson, the river that connects me to my childhood home of Albany. Then we fell asleep in each other's arms.

I woke in the middle of the night. I was lying on my back when I opened my eyes and there, suspended about an arm's length above my head was a bouquet of baby's breath floating in the air, as full, and white, and real as any I'd ever seen while wide awake. I could almost smell their fragrance.

I shook Mark's shoulder.

"What's wrong?" He sprang to attention, used to guarding me as he was.

"Nothing . . . but don't you see?"

He shook his head no.

"It's a fucking bouquet of baby's breath," I reported happily.

We laughed with relief—finally a joyful vision.

Unbeknownst to us, earlier that evening we'd conceived our daughter, Hannah Rose.

EPILOGUE

Soon after I started writing, I put away my early pages or turned them into fiction. For many years, the real story of my sleepwalking and sleep terrors was too personal to share beyond my circle of close friends and fellow artists. I was not as brave as my mentor would have me be.

Then, in 2010, I read the tragic story of Tobias Wong in the *New York Times*. He was a designer who had died at the age of thirty-five in what authorities ruled a suicide. Friends described him as an artist but not a tortured artist. They said that in the week before his death, he showed no signs of agitation or distress and seemed his normal self: upbeat, albeit with that familiar edge.

In private, Mr. Wong suffered from sleepwalking and sleep terrors. During episodes, he could perform elaborate tasks that required attention and concentration such as bill clients and make funny outfits for his cats. Once, while sleeping, he threw treasured artwork across the room, shattering the glass. Other times, he seemed panicked, as if fleeing an attacker. His partner of six years, Mr. Dubitsky, would sometimes find him incoherent and sobbing.

According to the article, Mr. Wong had no substance abuse issues or health problems, even though the point of the story was that severe, chronic sleepwalking probably led to his death. The *Times*, thankfully, printed a correction a week later: "As the article noted, he had a variety of sleep disorders, including chronic sleepwalking and sleep terrors; thus, it was not the case that he did not have a history of health problems."

I wonder, too, at another point made regarding this young man's mental health—"Unlike many Manhattanites, he wasn't even seeing a therapist." Does seeing a therapist mean that one has a problem, thereby if one doesn't see a therapist, one doesn't have a problem?

Apparently Mr. Wong met with countless doctors, although it is not reported if he saw a sleep specialist. Remedies he tried were listed: Ayurvedic diets, recordings of Tibetan singing bowls, sleeping pills—all unsuccessfully.

Mr. Dubitsky said that on the day of his partner's death, after dinner, they read, sent e-mail messages, then dozed off together on the couch. When he woke up a few hours later, Mr. Wong had slipped into a sleepwalking state. Mr. Dubitsky tried to chat with him, then went to bed. The next morning, he found his partner dead. The office of the chief medical examiner in Manhattan ruled it a suicide by hanging.

Dr. Mahowald was quoted, "Some sleepwalkers will go jogging on the freeway and be killed in traffic, or stroll off the deck of a cruise ship, unaware of their surroundings." He and fellow sleep specialists even coined the term *parasomnia pseudo-suicide*, in part because the fatalities are frequently misinterpreted.

Dr. Michel A. Cramer Bornemann, a colleague of Dr. Mahowald, said that the brain's prefrontal cortex is off-line in these cases. "That's important because that's where intent, awareness, and motivation resides," he said. "If that's not accessible, you don't have the awareness and motivation. So it's technically not suicide. It's an accident."

As I read the article, the paper shook in my hands. I wept for this young man and his loved ones. It could have been me. Mark held me as I confessed my last sleepwalking secret—the night of the open window. Even during all those years in therapy, I'd hidden the absolute truth of my near parasomnia pseudo-suicide.

I realized how selfish I'd been. It was time to share my story.

After suffering from sleepwalking and sleep terrors for twenty years, I have not suffered a violent episode of sleepwalking or sleep terrors in twenty-five years. My journey had taken place one night at a time. I never needed to go back on the Klonopin after the birth of my daughter but would not hesitate to do so if I had a recurrence.

What helps me sleep soundly is a combination of what worked for me at the start of my recovery and new efforts toward health along the way. I have a friend who says when we coast we have only one way to go—and that's downhill.

I've benefited over the years from: exercise (swimming, walking, dancing, and yoga); healthy eating, no caffeine or alcohol, avoiding sugar; practicing meditation and, very importantly, learning to understand and trust my intuition; therapy as needed; hypnosis and acupuncture; Eye Movement Desensitization and Reprocessing (EMDR)—a psychotherapy treatment that was originally designed to alleviate the distress associated with traumatic memories; Emotional Freedom Techniques (EFT)—a technique of tapping along the lines of the Chinese meridian system while simultaneously addressing emotional issues; wearing earplugs and an eye mask to bed; fun gatherings with friends; vibrant spiritual and artistic communities; quality time with loved ones; and, last but not least, avoiding the news, disturbing movies, and worrisome reading materials in the evening.

I'm fascinated by, in awe of, and tremendously appreciative of the advances in brain science, neuroscience, and sleep science of recent years. My healthful sleep is contingent upon maintenance of my emotional, spiritual, and physical wellness. The spiritual piece is, for me, extremely personal and equally mysterious. That's why when people ask, "How did you cure the sleepwalking and sleep terrors?" I see, mirrored in their faces, my own desire to control the uncontrollable. I see a longing for a simple solution.

My path to sound sleep was almost as mysterious as the sleepwalking and sleep terrors themselves.

It was a path back to myself.

APPENDIX

American Academy of Sleep Medicine: www.sleepeducation.com

American Society of Clinical Hypnosis: www.asch.net

Center for Advanced Research in Sleep Medicine

Dream and Nightmare Laboratory

Hôpital du Sacré-Coeur de Montréal: www.dreamscience.ca

National Institute of Mental Health: www.nimh.nih.gov

National Sleep Foundation: www.sleepfoundation.org

Sleep Forensic Associates: www.sleepforensicmedicine.org

Society of Behavioral Sleep Medicine (SBSM): www.behavioralsleep.org

World Association of Sleep Medicine: www.wasmonline.org

ARTICLES:

Baran A. S., Richert A. C., Goldberg R, Fry J. M. "Posttraumatic stress disorder in the spouse of a patient with sleep terrors." *Sleep Med.* 4 (2003): 73–75.

Cordi M. J., Schlarb A. A., Rasch B. "Deepening sleep by hypnotic suggestion." *Sleep* 52 (2014): 1143–52, 1152A–1152F.

Duval M., McDuff P., Zadra A. "Nightmare frequency, nightmare distress, and psychopathology in female victims of childhood maltreatment." *J Nerv Ment Dis.* 201 (2013): 767–72.

Finger S., Stiles A. "Lord Byron's physician: John William Polidori on somnambulism." *Prog Brain Res.* 205 (2013): 131–47.

Goldstein A. N., Greer S. M., Saletin J. M., Harvey A. G., Nitschke J. B., Walker M. P. "Tired and apprehensive: anxiety amplifies the impact of sleep loss on aversive brain anticipation." *J Neurosci* 33 (2013): 10607–15.

Gross C. R., Kreitzer M. J., Reilly-Spong M., Wall M., Winbush N. Y., Patterson R., Mahowald M., Cramer-Bornemann M. "Mindfulness-based stress reduction versus pharmacotherapy for chronic primary insomnia: a randomized controlled clinical trial." *Explore (NY)* 7 (2011): 76–87.

Kohler W. C., Kurz P. J., Kohler E. A. "A Case of Successful Use of Hypnosis in the Treatment of Parasomnia Overlap Disorder." *Behav Sleep Med.* 16 (April 2014): 1–10.

Leifker F. R., White K. H., Blandon A. Y., Marshall A. D. "Posttraumatic stress disorder symptoms impact the emotional experience of intimacy during couple discussions." *J Anxiety Disord.* 29C (2014): 119–127.

MacLehose W. "Sleepwalking, violence and desire in the middle ages." *Cult Med Psychiatry* 37 (2013): 601–24.

Mahowald M. W., Schenck C. H., Goldner M., Bachelder V., Cramer-Bornemann M. "Parasomnia pseudo-suicide." *J Forensic Sci.* 48 (2003): 1158–62.

Mahowald M. W., Schenck C. H. "Parasomnias: sleepwalking and the law." *Sleep Med Rev.* 4 (2000): 321–39.

Marshall A. J., Acheson D. T., Risbrough V. B., Straus L. D., Drummond S. P. "Fear conditioning, safety learning, and sleep in humans." *J Neurosci* 34 (2014): 11754–60.

Mysliwiec V., O'Reilly B., Polchinski J., Kwon H. P., Germain A., Roth B. J. "Trauma associated sleep disorder: a proposed parasomnia encompassing disruptive nocturnal behaviors, nightmares, and REM without atonia in trauma survivors." *J Clin Sleep Med.* 8 (2014): 1143–8.

Ohayon M. M., Mahowald M. W., Dauvilliers Y., et al. "Prevalence and comorbidity of nocturnal wandering in the U.S. adult general population." *Neurology* 78 (2012): 1583–9.

John M. Rumbold, M.B.Ch.B., Renata L. Riha, M.D., and Ian Morrison, Ph.D. "Alcohol and Non-Rapid Eye Movement Parasomnias: Where Is the Evidence?" *J Clin Sleep Med.* 10 (2014): 345.

Siclari F., Khatami R., Urbaniok F., Nobili L., Mahowald M. W., Schenck C. H., Cramer Bornemann M. A., Bassetti C. L. "Violence in sleep." *Brain* 133 (2010): 3494–509.

Szűcs A., Kamondi A., Zoller R., Barcs G., Szabó P., Purebl G. "Violent somnambulism: a parasomnia of young men with stereotyped dream-like experiences." *Med Hypotheses* 83 (2014): 47–52.

Walker M. P., van der Helm E. "Overnight therapy? The role of sleep in emotional brain processing." *Psychol Bull.* 135 (2009): 731–48.

Wolke D., Lereya S. T. "Bullying and parasomnias: a longitudinal cohort study." *Pediatrics* 134 (2014): e1040–8.

Zadra A., Desautels A., Petit D., Montplaisir J. "Somnambulism: clinical aspects and pathophysiological hypotheses." *Lancet Neurol.* 12 (2013): 85–94.

BOOKS:

International Classification of Sleep Disorders: Diagnostic & Coding Manual Paperback by American Academy of Sleep Medicine
Publisher: American Academy of Sleep Medicine 2005
ISBN-10: 0965722023
ISBN-13: 978-0965722025

Sleepwalk with Me: and Other Painfully True Stories by Mike Birbiglia
Publisher: Simon & Schuster 2012
ISBN-10: 1439157995
ISBN-13: 978-1439157992

The Twenty-four Hour Mind: The Role of Sleep and Dreaming in Our Emotional Lives by Rosalind D. Cartwright
Publisher: Oxford University Press 2012
ISBN-10: 0199896283
ISBN-13: 978-0199896288

Food and Healing by Annemarie Colbin
Publisher: Ballantine Books 1986
ISBN-10: 0345303857
ISBN-13: 978-0345303851

The Brain That Changes Itself: Stories of Personal Triumph from the Frontiers of Brain Science by Norman Doidge M.D

Publisher: Penguin Books 2007
ISBN-10: 0143113100
ISBN-13: 978-0143113102

Shattered Assumptions (Towards a New Psychology of Trauma) by Ronnie
Janoff-Bulman
Waking the Tiger: Healing Trauma by Peter A. Levine
Publisher: North Atlantic Books 2002
ISBN-10: 155643233X
ISBN-13: 978-1556432330

Dreamland: Adventures in the Strange Science of Sleep by David K. Randall
Publisher: W. W. Norton & Company 2013
ISBN-10: 0393345866
ISBN-13: 978-0393345865

The Body Remembers: The Psychophysiology of Trauma and Trauma Treatment
(Norton Professional Book) by Babette Rothschild
Publisher: W. W. Norton & Company 2002
ISBN-10: 0393703274
ISBN-13: 978-0393703276

*Getting Past Your Past: Take Control of Your Life with Self-Help Techniques from
EMDR Therapy* by Francine Shapiro
Publisher: Rodale Books 2013
ISBN-10: 1609619951
ISBN-13: 978-1609619954

Stalking Irish Madness: Searching for the Roots of My Family's Schizophrenia by
Patrick Tracey
Publisher: Bantam 2008
ISBN-10: 0553805258
ISBN-13: 978-0553805253

The Body Keeps the Score: Brain, Mind, and Body in the Healing of Trauma
by Bessel van der Kolk MD
Publisher: Viking Adult 2014
ISBN-10: 0670785938
ISBN-13: 978-0670785933

ACKNOWLEDGMENTS

Heartfelt thanks to the early supporters at The Actors Studio: Ellen Burstyn, Terese Hayden, Jacqueline Brooks, Vivian Nathan, Dina Janis, Jacqueline Knapp, and Norman Mailer. Appreciation to my agent, Jill Marsal, likewise to Nicole Frail, Tony Lyons, and everyone at Skyhorse Publishing. Gratitude to my stalwart cohorts: Newelle MacDonald, Tom Fuld and Kaelin Fuld, Julie Boak and David Irons, Carroll Terry, Barbara Suter, Sue Shapiro, Dianne and Andy Marino, JoD Andrews and family, Maureen Throp and Dale Rutkin; A Dance for All Peoples, especially Clyde Hall, Laine Thom, Charles Lawrence, Ann Roberts, Joan Henry, Nancy Martinez, Charlie Patton, Barbara Snyder, Deborah Wolf, Murray Edelman, Lucy West, Hollis Melton, Robert Sink, Ted Welch, Tony Allicino, Ron Madson, Franklin Coursin, Constance Rodgers, Robert Croonquist, Margaret Downing Dill, Sean Dill, Elias Guerrero, and Michael Picucci; Regena Thomashauer, The School of Womanly Arts, Sheila Hay, Jennifer Terrell, Ann Moller, Lori Sutherland, and Tracy Marx; Angelo Verga and The Cornelia Street Cafe; my writers' groups over the years and especially the Ninety-Sixth Street gang; all the folks at *Psychology Today*; The Norman Mailer Center; Malachy McCourt, Peter Quinn, Mary Pat Kelly, Larry Kirwan, Seamus Scanlon, and Irish American Writers and Artists; Charles Hale and Artists Without Walls; the Narrative Medicine Literature Study Group at Columbia

University Medical Center; my health care practitioners, in particular Annie Fox, Neila Wyman and Drs. Neil Kavey, Michael Borecky, Robert Schiller; Dr. Mark Mahowald for his foreword; with love to my parents for their heroic efforts toward health, to my almitas, to my beloved siblings, to Joe and Carol Dahm and their brood; dear appreciation to Zach and Hannah; finally, in gratitude to my husband, Mark Dahm, without whose friendship this book would not have been possible, and whose love and gentleness have gifted me with many peaceful nights' slumber.